Craniofacial Deformities

D.J. David D.C. Hemmy R.D. Cooter

Craniofacial Deformities

Atlas of Three-Dimensional Reconstruction from Computed Tomography

With 106 Illustrations in 461 Parts

Springer-Verlag
New York Berlin Heidelberg
London Paris Tokyo Hong Kong

David J. David, MBBS, FRACS, Director
The Australian Craniofacial Unit, Adelaide Children's Hospital, Inc.,
North Adelaide, South Australia 5006

David C. Hemmy, MD, FACS
Professor, Departments of Neurosurgery and Plastic Surgery,
Director, Craniofacial Research, Medical College of Wisconsin,
Milwaukee, Wisconsin 52336, USA

Rodney D. Cooter, MBBS
The Australian Craniofacial Unit, Adelaide Children's Hospital, Inc.,
North Adelaide, South Australia 5006

The *cover* represents a composite of images. Those on the left were obtained from a near-perfect edition of Andreas Vesalius' *Fabrica* (1543) housed in the History of Medicine collection of the Todd Wehr Libraries of the Medical College of Wisconsin. The drawings presented in this work were painstakingly rendered from anatomical dissections of the bodies of criminals. The images on the right were acquired and rendered electronically without invasion of the body. These images can be had within minutes of acquisition. Virtually no artist's license is permitted in the electronic image such that, although the images are extremely faithful, the presentation may not match that of Vesalius more than 400 years ago.

Library of Congress Cataloging-in-Publication Data
David, David John, 1940–
Craniofacial deformities.
Includes bibliographies.
1. Face—Abnormalities—Atlases. 2. Face—Tomography—Atlases. 3. Skull—Abnormalities—Atlases. 4. Skull—Tomography—Atlases. 5. Three-dimensional display systems. I. Hemmy, David C. II. Cooter, R. D. (Rodney D.) III. Title. [DNLM: 1. Facial Bones—abnormalities—atlases. 2. Facial Bones—injuries—atlases. 3. Image Processing, Computer-Assisted—atlases. 4. Skull—abnormalities—atlases. 5. Skull—injuries—atlases. WE 17 D249c]
QM695.F32D38 1989 617'.52'0022 89-4263

Typeset by Bi-Comp, Inc., York, Pennsylvania.
Printed and bound by Arcata Graphics/Halliday, West Hanover, Massachusetts.
Printed in the United States of America.

9 8 7 6 5 4 3 2 1

ISBN 0-387-96969-1 Springer-Verlag New York Berlin Heidelberg
ISBN 3-540-96969-1 Springer-Verlag Berlin Heidelberg New York

Preface

This book has been assembled from the radiographic and photographic records of patients presenting to craniofacial units on four continents over 7 years. It is our purpose to illustrate a wide range of craniofacial deformities with the technique of three-dimensional computed tomography. Many topics are briefly addressed with descriptive text intended to amplify the accompanying images but not to exclude the need for more comprehensive references as recommended in the reading list of each chapter.

The ability to generate three-dimensional radiographic images represents a successful integration of computed tomography with computer graphics. Although this technique remains an electronic substitute for the study of dry skull specimens, it offers a permanent pictorial record of anatomical structures with the opportunity for future interactive data manipulation.

It is hoped, therefore, that this work will assist others to gain a more complete understanding of disorders of the craniofacial region. We encourage other surgeons and investigators to examine and employ the techniques used to gather these images but also to ensure that standardized scanning regimens are adapted. The importance of data collection within its full anatomical context was borne out with many of our early studies, which were limited owing to computational constraints. Often an image requirement for surgical intervention is much less than an image necessary for strict scientific inquiry. Furthermore, we believe that permanent data storage is imperative for future analyses and that optimal use can be made of data stored in its initial slice format.

Adelaide, Australia, and
Milwaukee, Wisconsin, USA

David J. David
David C. Hemmy
Rodney D. Cooter

Acknowledgments

We thank Professor Gabor T. Herman whose technology made possible this exciting method of study. Dr. Thomas Lindquist of Dimensional Medicine, Incorporated, provided technical advice and adapted his skills to our requirements in the preparation of a work station. We thank Drs. Bruce Clark, Lloyd Morris, Lance Perrett, and Alan Williams for their patience and cooperation with our use of their CT facilities. Graham Truman, Marion Tregeagle, and Amanda Sierp of the Adelaide Children's Hospital, Department of Radiology, performed most of the superb studies and attended to the minute details of CT data collection; this work is gratefully acknowledged. The photography and illustrations of Mark Stevens, Alex Sukys, Christopher Sprod, Jan Nicol, and Colleen Lloyd stand on the following pages as examples of their expertise. We are also grateful to Dr. Amanda Abbott, Marika Cummings, Lea Frick, Mary Thielke, Kim Goncalves, Amanda Borg-Cardona, Judith Walker, Carole Graff, Rachel David, and Kirsten Hemmy for their effort in attending to detail, both major and minor, in the preparation of this atlas.

We hope that this work will illustrate our gratitude to computer scientists for developing the technique of three-dimensional imaging, which has provided us with a greater insight into craniofacial disorders.

Contents

1

History of Three-Dimensional Imaging of Craniofacial Disorders

The ultimate understanding of the deranged anatomical state is derived by studying postmortem specimens. However, the craniofacial disorders, which are rare and predominantly nonfatal, provide a paucity of material for collection, study, and classification. Investigation of craniofacial disorders must then, by necessity, be directed to the living patient using the investigative tools at hand (chiefly noninvasive but occasionally invasive), relying on limited intraoperative photography and the keen memory of the surgeon.

Since the time of Roentgen we have been able to delineate the macroscopic structure of hidden organs. The two-dimensional superimposition of organs using standard x-ray techniques results in anatomical obscuration of both normal and pathological structures, limiting the accuracy of this modality. The use of polytomography, which requires that the tube and cassette move about the patient as well as the addition of contrast agents, aids in distinguishing one structure from another. However, these methods still fall prey to the valid criticisms of lack of tridimensionality (as one perceives objects in the surrounding milieu by means of binocular vision) and necessary interpretation by an experienced individual. Furthermore, interpretations are recorded verbally, are often imprecise, and vary from observation to observation.

The introduction of computed tomography (CT) by Hounsfield in 1973 provided a sophisticated method for examining the internal structure of the body on a macroscopic level without obscuration by overlapping structures. Computed tomograms provide information about "slices" of the human body. If the CT slices are obtained in an abutting or overlapping fashion, a set of measurements are obtained that, if displayed correctly, can provide three-dimensional anatomical information. This fact was first recognized by Herman and Liu in 1977.

Hemmy et al. suggested in 1979 that rendered three-dimensional images would be useful to the understanding of pediatric craniofacial and spinal anomalies. They believed that the three-dimensional image stood as a permanent graphic assembly of CT slice data in contradistinction to the often erroneous mental assimilation and reconstruction of multiple CT slices, which also has the disadvantage of error among interpreters.

The method of Gabor Herman was introduced to the South Australian Craniofacial Unit by David Hemmy in 1980. The introduction was met with some skepticism, as technically sophisticated polytomographic equipment was already situated and used by the group at Adelaide Children's Hospital. Furthermore, the large-aperture, high-resolution scanner was just being introduced. The nearest site capable of providing this service was Hobart, Tasmania—well over 1100 kilometers away. Nonetheless, through research funding and persistence, several patients were scanned in Hobart. Image processing, limited in the number of slices that could be processed and therefore incapable of presenting the full anatomical context, was carried out at the State University of New York in Buffalo in the laboratories of Gabor Herman. Technical problems were solved by long distance telephone. Needless to say, a considerable time elapsed between scanning and presentation of the rendered images in Adelaide (Fig. 1.1). In a few cases, the images arrived after the surgery had been completed. In addition to the great physical distances involved in this project, image processing was slow, requiring 8–12 hours for batch image processing.

Over the next year the utility of the three-dimensional presentation of CT data was realized. Confidence in the accuracy of the image as well as the usefulness of having available a nearly infinite number of possible views served to eliminate polytomography as a major investigative tool. By 1982, CT and reconstructed views were the major radiographic tool at the South Australian Craniofacial Unit. Reconstruction of three-dimensional data was carried out for two more years as an experimental protocol at the laboratories of David Hemmy. In 1984, commercial prototype software became available, making the Adelaide unit self-sufficient.

By 1983, case material had been collected and examined and the clinical efficacy determined. Publications by Hemmy et al. (1983) and Marsh and Vannier (1983) attested to the usefulness of this modality. Both of these clinical reports used a three-dimensional display similar to the method of Herman and Udupa (1981). By this time three-dimensional display of craniofacial data was routine at the Medical College of Wisconsin, the South Australian Craniofacial Unit, and Washington University (St. Louis).

Computed tomography and the reconstruction of CT data in three dimensions has, over a period of 7 years, completely eliminated many conventional radiographic examinations and now is beginning to seriously threaten radiocephalometry. The recent reduction in the cost of both hardware and software systems supporting three-dimensional reconstruction makes these systems an economic reality.

Recommended Reading

Hemmy DC, David DJ, Herman GT: Three dimensional reconstruction of craniofacial deformity using computed tomography. Neurosurgery 13:534–541, 1983.

Hemmy DC, Herman GT, Millar EA, Haughton VM: Three-dimensional reconstruction of the spine and calvarium in children utilizing computed tomography. In: Proceedings of the Second International Child Neurology Congress, Sydney, Australia, p 81, 1979.

Herman GT, Liu HK: Display of three-dimensional information in computed tomography. J Comput Assist Tomogr 1:155–160, 1977.

Herman GT, Udupa JK: Display of three-dimensional discrete surfaces. Proc SPIE 283:90–97, 1981.

Hokayem N: The investigation and information drawn from dry skulls. In Caronni EP (ed): Craniofacial Surgery. Little, Brown, Boston, p 12, 1985.

Hounsfield GN: Computerized transverse axial scanning (tomography). I. Description of the system. Br J Radiol 46:1016–1022, 1973.

Marsh JL, Vannier MW: The "third" dimension in craniofacial surgery. Plast Reconstr Surg 71:759–767, 1983.

Tessier PL, Hemmy DC: 3-D imaging in medicine . . . a critique by surgeons. Scand J Plast Reconstr Surg 20:3–11, 1986.

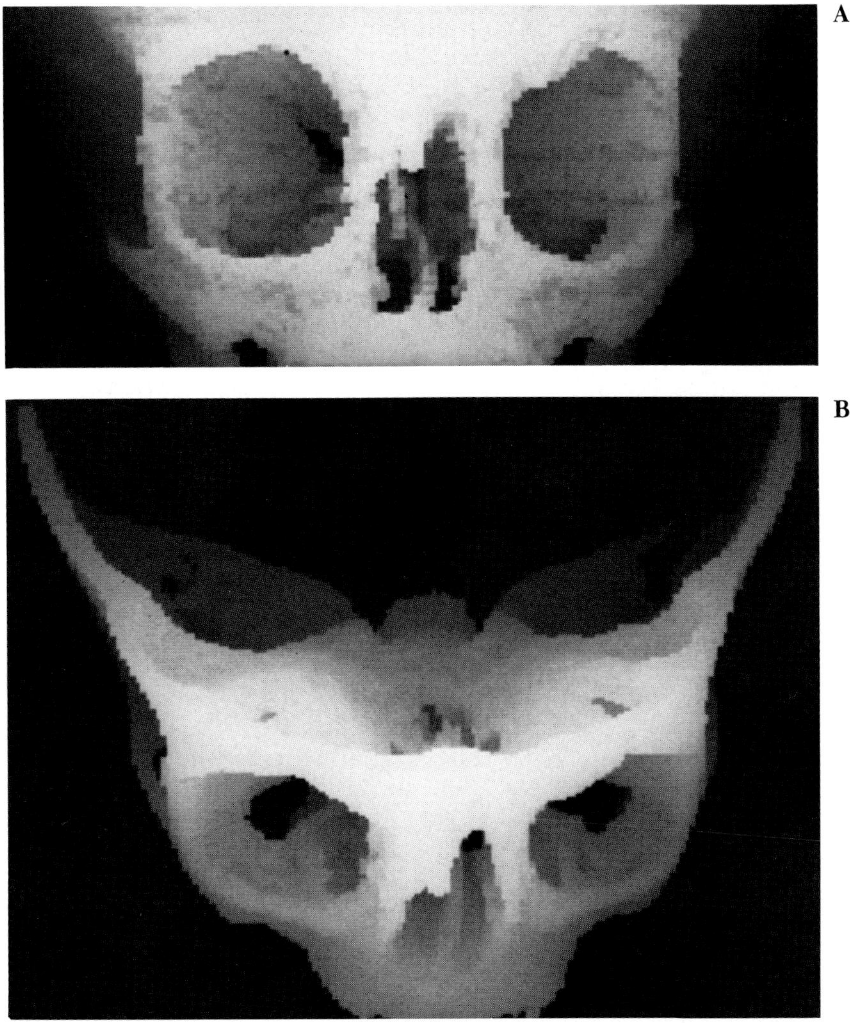

Fig. 1.1. Three-dimensional image of patient with midfacial cleft and orbital hypertelorism acquired in Hobart, processed in Buffalo, and used in Adelaide.

C

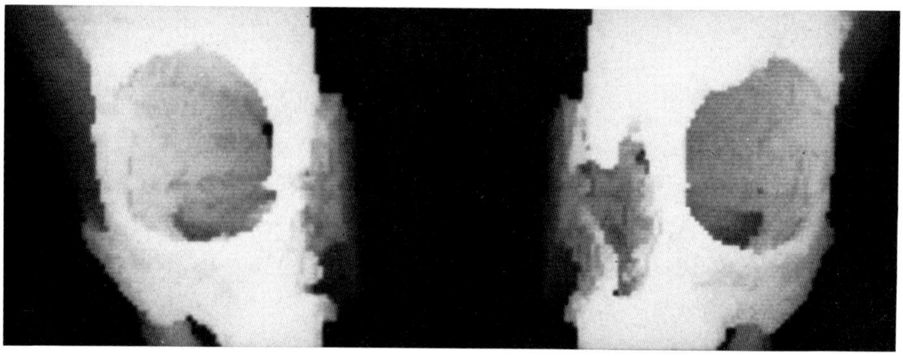

D

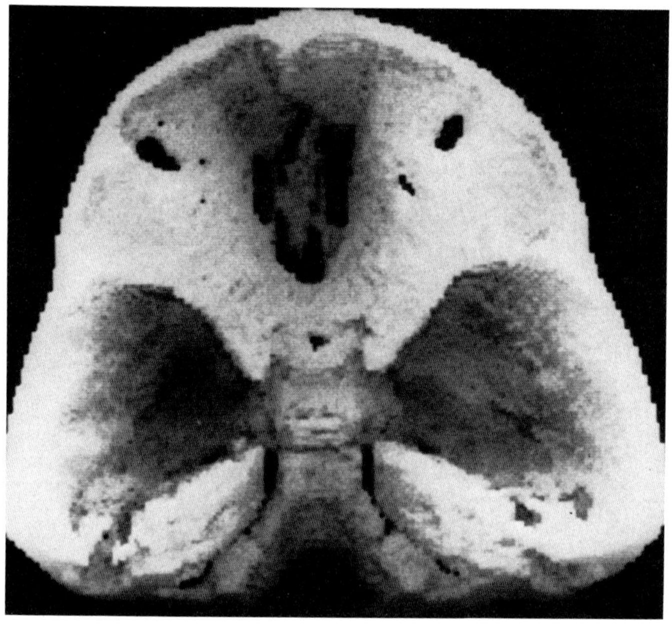

Fig. 1.1 (contd)

2

Three-Dimensional Imaging Techniques

Currently, there are a number of software programs designed to provide three-dimensional reformatting of computed tomography (CT) and to operate on computer equipment supplied with CT acquisition systems. These programs, unless operating on an independent work station, are subordinate to the reconstruction programs necessary for slice display. This method facilitates handling of the great volume of data to be processed. Consequently, when reference is made to a work station, it is a dedicated work station, currently the IIS (Dimensional Medicine, Inc., Minnetonka, Minnesota).

Generation of a three-dimensional image may be divided into a number of steps, including CT scanning, data selection, and data processing.

CT Scanning

It must be emphasized a priori that the acquisition and production of a high quality, high fidelity three-dimensional study begins with scrupulous attention to detail. It is important that the personnel of the radiology department understand the purpose of the study, with stress placed on the fact that these studies are used to comprehend, with great detail, anatomical variance rather than to make a diagnosis or place a particular pathology "label" on the anomaly. With this requirement in mind, the wishes of the surgeon (which sometimes seem excessive to the radiologist) are followed.

The patient must remain motionless during the study. It is an absolute requirement such that the patient should be sedated or anesthetized. To date, there is no easy correction for misregistration of CT slices. The patient's head is restrained in a head holder with the orbitomeatal line perpendicular to the floor.

The surgeon designates the area to be scanned (Fig. 2.1). Ideally, this information is conveyed to the radiographer by means of a drawing or marks on a photograph of the patient. The areas of extreme interest are scanned, obtaining the thinnest slices possible (usually 1.5 mm), whereas areas of lesser interest but necessary to provide an anatomical context are scanned to allow a slice thickness of 3–5 mm (Fig. 2.2). The ordinary craniofacial study requires 100–150 slices.

Optimum scan factors should include the soft tissue technique (particularly the first time a patient is scanned) to highlight associated soft tissue anomalies, an image matrix of 512 × 512, and a narrow field of view. Using a phantom we have determined that, provided abutting (rather than overlapping) slices are used, the total radiation delivered to the area scanned is, at maximum, 5 rad, as the x-ray beam is tightly collimated. Although newer programs permit correction for tilt of the CT gantry, tilting should be avoided unless it is necessary to avoid the inaccuracies produced from metallic dental restorations or appliances. Lastly, a reasonable amount of time (45–75 minutes) should be set aside for the scan. Nearly all problems result from a poorly performed scan.

Data Selection

Data selection implies an observer interaction. CT slices are reviewed sequentially, if necessary. Slices at either extreme of the sequence may be rejected if they are not germane to reconstruction. Because the CT slices are composed of picture elements (*pixels*) having gray values proportional to the attenuation of the x-ray beam by the tissue represented, and because the three-dimensional object is to be a "dissection" of the object scanned, tissues or gray values must be removed through a process called *segmentation*, or *thresholding*, in order that only the values of interest are included. Furthermore, by a process called *subregioning*, only those areas of the entire CT slice that are of interest are selected for economy of computation. At this time, if the surgeon has a protocol of predetermined views, or "pose angles," only those views of interest are selected.

Threshold selection is an important step. There is a reasonable amount of information loss, both intentional and unintentional, that occurs between acquisition of the CT scan and provision of the rendered three-dimensional image (Fig. 2.3). Incorrect thresholding can render the displayed image inaccurate, permitting the inclusion or exclusion of data and causing a false representation (Fig. 2.4).

Image Processing

It is necessary to obtain a natural and correct perception of the full three-dimensional spatial relations of often complex patient anatomy. As noted, the processing of a set of original CT images into a rendered three-dimensional image (or a pseudo three-dimensional object) typically removes a significant amount of information. There is the possibility that this gain in perception may introduce some ambiguity. Therefore certain image criteria must be met to satisfy clinical criteria.

A number of alternative models for generating a two-dimensional image of a three-dimensional object may be considered. In essence, such models define how a final image is to be formed, typically by simulating transmission and reflection of light by objects of interest. One possible approach is to generate an image in which the brightness of a pixel is related to the total thickness of the object along a given ray (such as a transmission radiograph). This approach, however, is insensitive to surface irregularities, which may be clinically important. Accordingly, we use the alternative of computing rendered images based on a surface shading model. With this approach, the brightness of a pixel is based on computation of diffusely reflected light from the surface, which depends on both the depth of a surface element (*surfel*) and its attitude (*surface normal direction*) with respect to the incident light and viewing directions (Fig. 2.5).

The surface shading approach permits varying the number and location of simulated light sources that can be used and the rate at which reflected brightness may drop off with increasing depth and angles of incidence and reflection of the light. Using interactive control of surface normal and depth shading along with arbitrary three-axis rotations permits subtle details to be seen.

The image quality of shaded surface images is affected by the relative strengths of the depth shading and surface normal shading. Although to some extent the judging of these images is a subjective matter, those images that are relatively restricted in their edge darkening are most suitable for anatomical display.

Occasionally it is desirable to view more than one surface at a time. In such cases, multiple surfaces can be exhibited using transparency and color to facilitate viewing (Fig. 2.6).

Typical computer graphics methods fit curves or patches to relatively sparsely defined data and subsequently render images from these smooth curves or patches. However, high resolution CT data are far from sparsely defined; moreover, a fracture or foramen as narrow as one pixel in a 512 × 512 image matrix may be clinically significant, requiring that it be visible on the final image. Therefore a volume element (*voxel*) data representation making use of a regular three-dimensional array called a *binary volume* is used. The binary volume has a granularity that is typically less than the size of the resolution elements of the original data and is not based on any assumptions of object smoothness, orientation, or the contiguous relations of elements, called *connectivity*. This representation simply assigns a binary value of 1 to each element included after segmentation or thresholding and a binary value of 0 to elements not fulfilling the criterion.

In many cases of clinical importance, segmentation is normally accomplished by applying a threshold criterion to the original CT pixel values. Pixel values between specified minimum and maximum values are considered "bone" and are assigned a binary value of 1. In most of these cases, the object contrast and signal-to-noise ratio are high, requiring no special data preparation or conditioning prior to thresholding. In certain scanned areas where representative tissues are thin or small and surrounded by tissues that have markedly different CT values (e.g., ethmoid bone and the air-containing sinus), the reconstructed CT image presents a third value (*partial volume average*) not representative of either tissue. Thresholding procedures applied to this value result, generally, in exclusion of bone in the rendered object, giving the appearance of a hole where one, in actuality, does not exist. In order to avoid these errors, two-dimensional image processing can be applied to the original CT slices to enhance some characteristic prior to segmentation. A problem seen with "dropout" of the ethmoid bone in many of the earlier images can now be corrected by applying a combined linear and nonlinear filter to enhance the thin bone without increasing background noise (which could be included as "bone" and therefore cause an error in appearance) (Fig. 2.7).

Prior to computing an binary value for the original CT pixel values based on thresholding, it is often appropriate to compute interpolated pixel values on a three-dimensional mesh of points that provides even finer spacing than the original pixel data. It provides a voxel (like a pixel, a voxel has an X and a Y dimension, but because it is a volume element it also has a third, or Z, dimension) smaller than the original data resolution element dimensions (Fig. 2.8). No error is created, as this interpolation does not add information to the original data but simply allows the original gray scale pixel data to be optimally used. It is clear that fidelity in the rendered images requires at least as many voxels as there were pixels in the original CT data. Consider CT data consisting of individual slices formed with a pixel matrix of 512 × 512 (512 rows of pixels and 512 columns of pixels). One hundred contiguous slices have been obtained, which results in a voxel volume of 512 × 512 × 100 voxels. After thresholding is applied, a binary volume is created that has these same dimensions (512 × 512 × 100). Interpolating these data could result in a binary volume having dimensions of 1000 × 1000 × 1000 elements or 512 × 512 × 512 elements. Not surprisingly, there is not a significant difference in the final rendered images using these two volumes, as resolution of the original 512 × 512 × 100 data presents the same fundamental limitations in both cases.

Gabor Herman and the Medical Image Processing Group presently located at the University of Pennsylvania developed an algorithm for computing a boundary surface comprised of voxel faces that are interfaces between 1 (present) and 0 (not present) voxels; they are mutually connected and also connected to a user-prescribed "seed point" on the boundary surface of interest. This technique uses connectivity criteria to build six lists of voxel surface elements, which correspond to the six possible directions of a voxel face (a voxel being a parallelepiped, which may be cubic). An important characteristic of this algorithm is that objects not connected to the surface of interest are automatically eliminated, a feature of utility in the elimination of an extraneous object of bone density such as the head holder or tape applied to the patient's forehead. A drawback to this processing method is the possible exclusion of anatomical parts that are not connected to one another, such as a bone sequestrum or the parietal bone as a portion of the skull in an infant.

A second surface extraction algorithm, not based on connectivity of voxels is also available. This method is several times faster than the connectivity method and is capable of handling large binary volumes (1000 × 1000 × 1000), as random access to the entire volume at once is not required. This method has the limitation that unwanted objects, such as the CT head holder, must be removed or "disarticulated" by the operator. However, disconnected portions of bone are always faithfully represented. Furthermore, "neighbor" codes, which define the orientation of the four faces connected to the displayed voxel face, are not generated, which affects some of the shading algorithms.

When a voxel surface has been generated by either of the methods, its elements (surfels) are projected onto a display matrix. The work station uses a depth buffer algorithm that, in a given display pixel, retains only the projected surfel that comes closest to the viewer. A surfel is projected orthographically into only those pixels whose centers lie within the bounds of the projected surfel.

Shading of the object can be based on surface neighbor codes (if a seed point has been defined) or on gradients in the depth image generated during projection into the display space. In the case of gradient shading, a small modulation from the discrete projected voxel face orientations is retained to provide the viewer with a subtle contouring effect, which serves as a depth cue. Using either the neighbor code-based or gradient-based choices for image rendering, the operator may select the relative amount of depth shading and surface normal shading to be used (Fig. 2.9).

The dedicated work station offers flexibility in the design of the anatomical object to be displayed. An "interactive" mode permits arbitrary three-axis rotation of the object. Furthermore, the permitted use of one or two binary volumes and a third "gray" volume containing complete 12-bit original pixel data permits internal inspection of an object from any desired viewpoint, displaying soft tissue alongside bone (Fig. 2.10).

Measurements can be made by determining three-dimensional coordinates (because there is a unique depth coordinate for the most frontal voxel along any ray). The distance between these coordinates can easily be computed and displayed. The definition of three consecutive points permits angular determination at the second, or vertex, point. Furthermore, volumetric measurements can be made by assessing the number of voxels contained in a defined space and converting this total to cubic centimeters (Fig. 2.11).

Work Station

The speed required for interactive three-dimensional image processing is provided by a flexible image/graphics processing "engine," which works in conjunction with its own high speed memory, and a "supermicro" UNIX based host computer, which is coupled to the interactive devices ("mouse" and trackball) of the work station. The database is stored on two large-capacity Winchester disks. The work station in a large craniofacial unit is a surgical tool dedicated to the tasks of the unit, permitting day-to-day image processing dictated by the case load of the unit as well as investigative study of the collected cases of the unit (Figs. 2.12–2.15).

Work Station Products

The permanent record of work station production comprises rendered images stored on a selected type of medium. That medium may be magnetic tape in the form of a video tape record of manipulation of images that occurred during the work session. It may also take a form suitable for storage and later review of archived images on magnetic tape suitable for review on the work station. Images may be captured by means of a 35-mm camera to record output. An experimental mode of transmission of images to a remote electronic terminal is also in evolution. Lastly, the most common form of work product is presently displayed on transparency film using a laser imager (Fig. 2.16). This medium has the advantage of portability.

Recommended Reading

Hemmy DC, Tessier PL: CT of dry skulls with craniofacial deformities: accuracy of three-dimensional reconstruction. Radiology 157:113–116, 1985.

Hemmy DC, Tessier PL, David DJ: Methods for and pitfalls in the acquisition of computed tomographic data for faithful three-dimensional reconstructions. In Marchac D (ed): Craniofacial Surgery (pp. 9–11). Springer-Verlag, Berlin, 1987.

Herman GT, Udupa JK: Display of three-dimensional discrete surfaces. Proc SPIE 283:90–97, 1981.

Tessier PL, Hemmy DC: 3-D Imaging in medicine . . . a critique by surgeons. Scand J Plast Reconstr Surg 20:3–11, 1986.

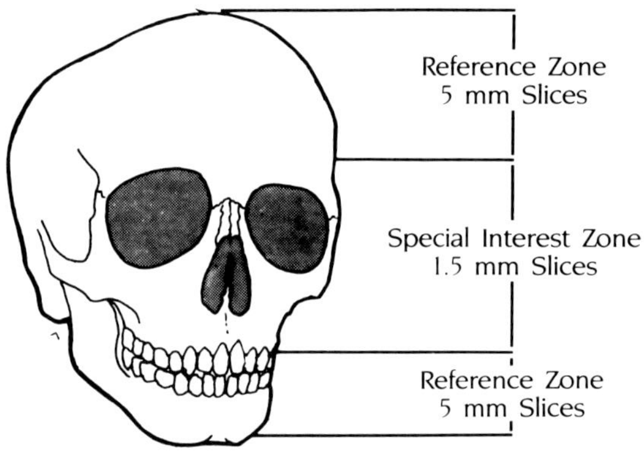

Fig. 2.1. Method of specifying CT scans with thin slices in the area of interest and thicker slices in reference area or area of anatomical context.

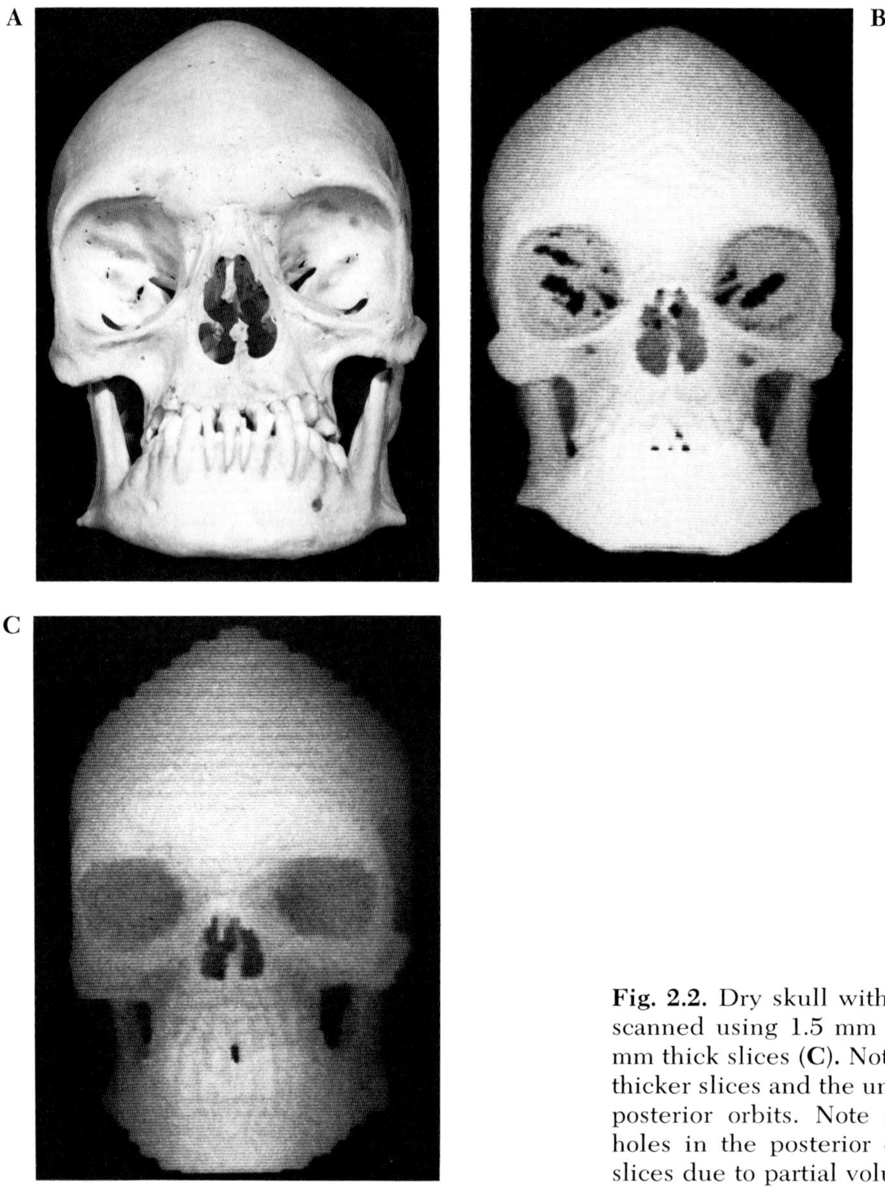

Fig. 2.2. Dry skull with Crouzon syndrome (**A**) scanned using 1.5 mm thick slices (**B**) and 5.0 mm thick slices (**C**). Note the lack of detail with thicker slices and the uniform appearance of the posterior orbits. Note also the appearance of holes in the posterior orbits on 1.5 mm thick slices due to partial volume averaging.

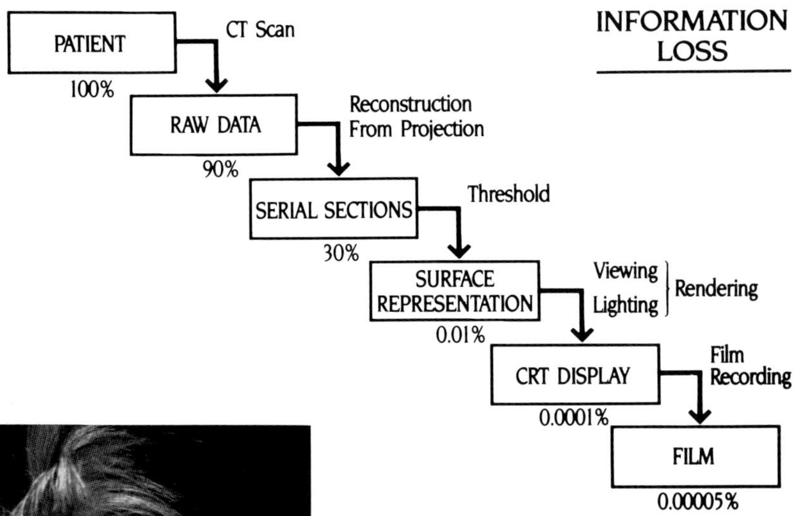

A

B

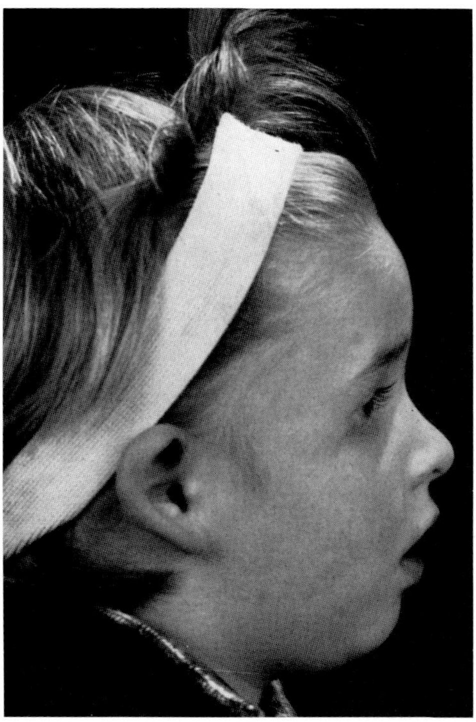

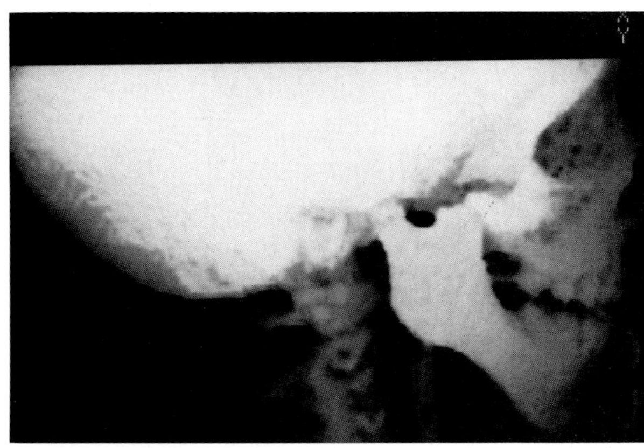

C

Fig. 2.3. Sequential map of information loss (**A**) that may occur from acquisition of data from patient (**B**) to rendered image (**C**). [(**A**) From Michael Vannier, MD, Mallinckrodt Institute, St. Louis, MO.]

A

B

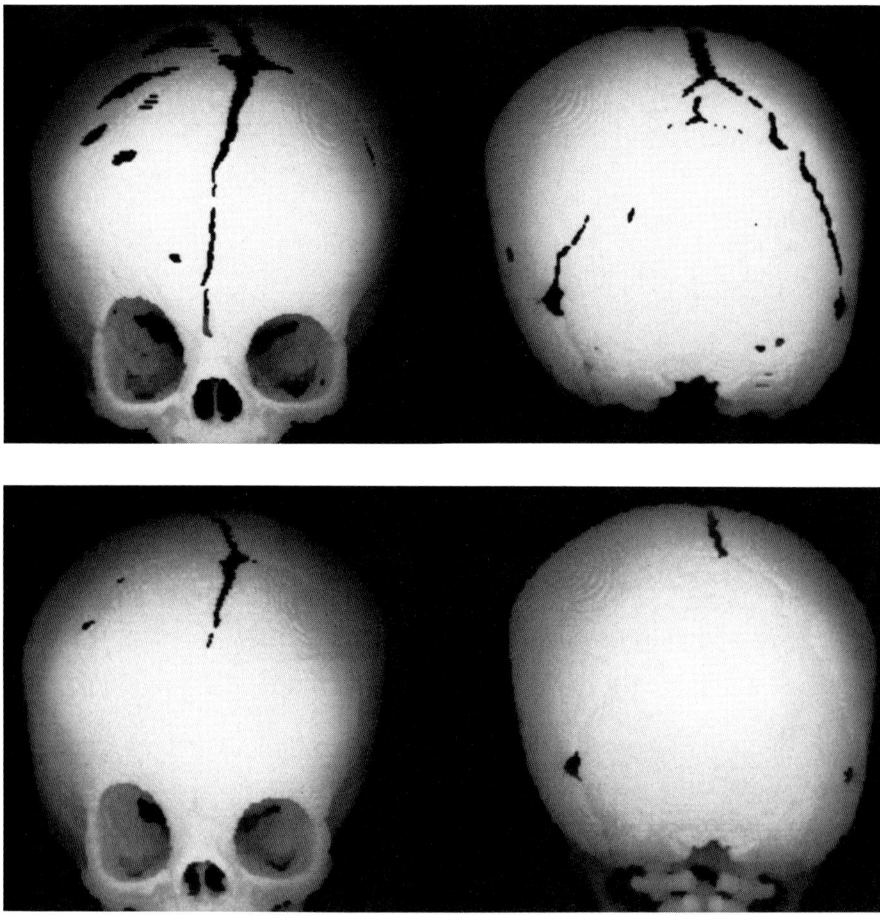

Fig. 2.4. Error that may occur because of incorrect threshold. **A** Incorrect image. **B** Correct image.

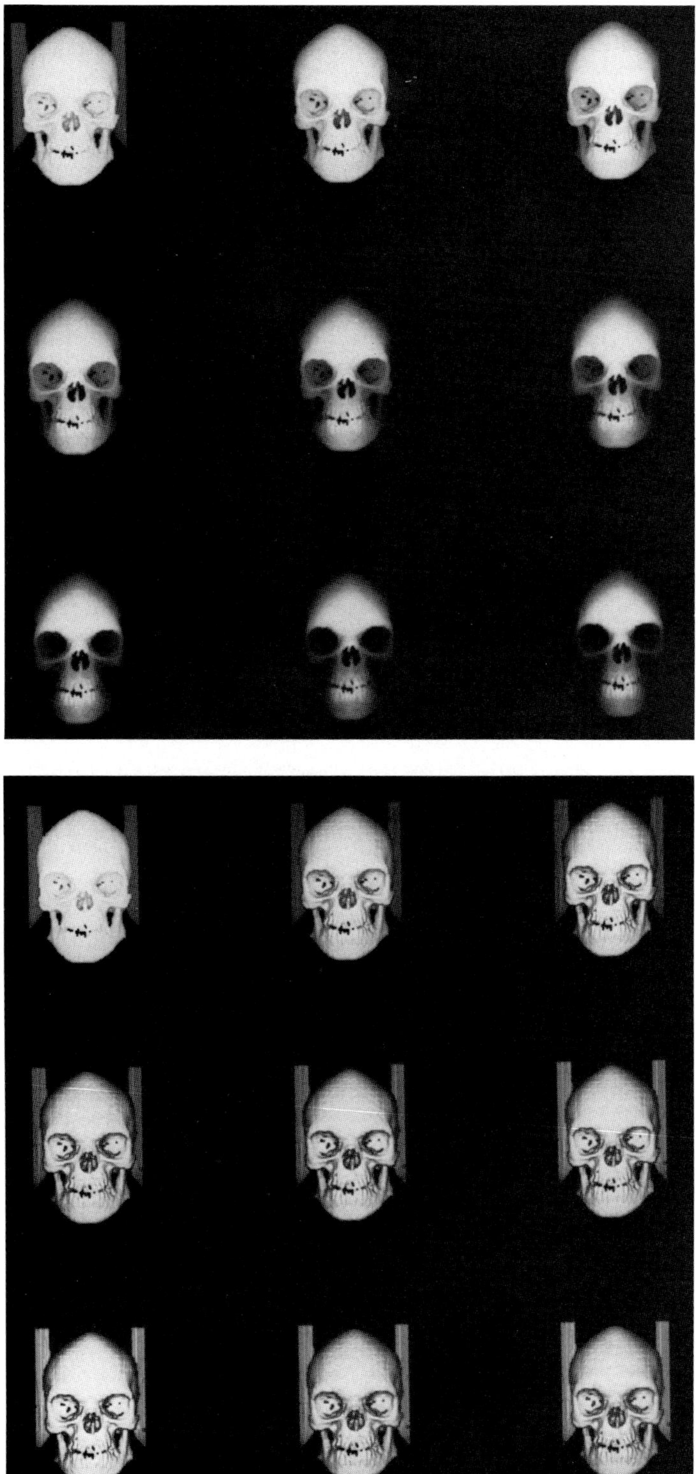

A

B

Fig. 2.5. A Images resulting from changes in depth shading. **B** Images resulting from changes in surface normal shading.

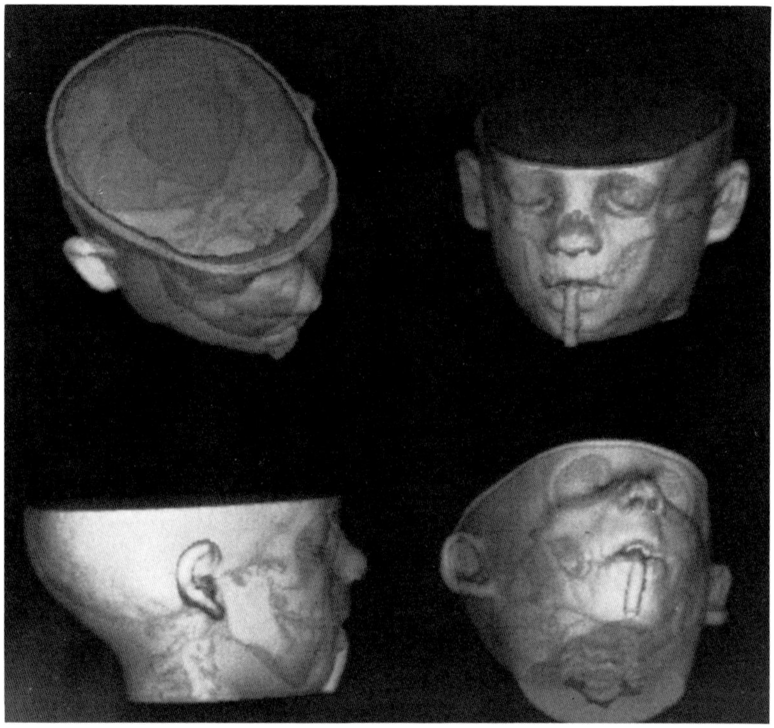

Fig. 2.6. Image created using transparency for simultaneous display of two tissues.

Fig. 2.8. Images resulting from use of voxels ▶ larger (**A**) and smaller (**B**) than original data.

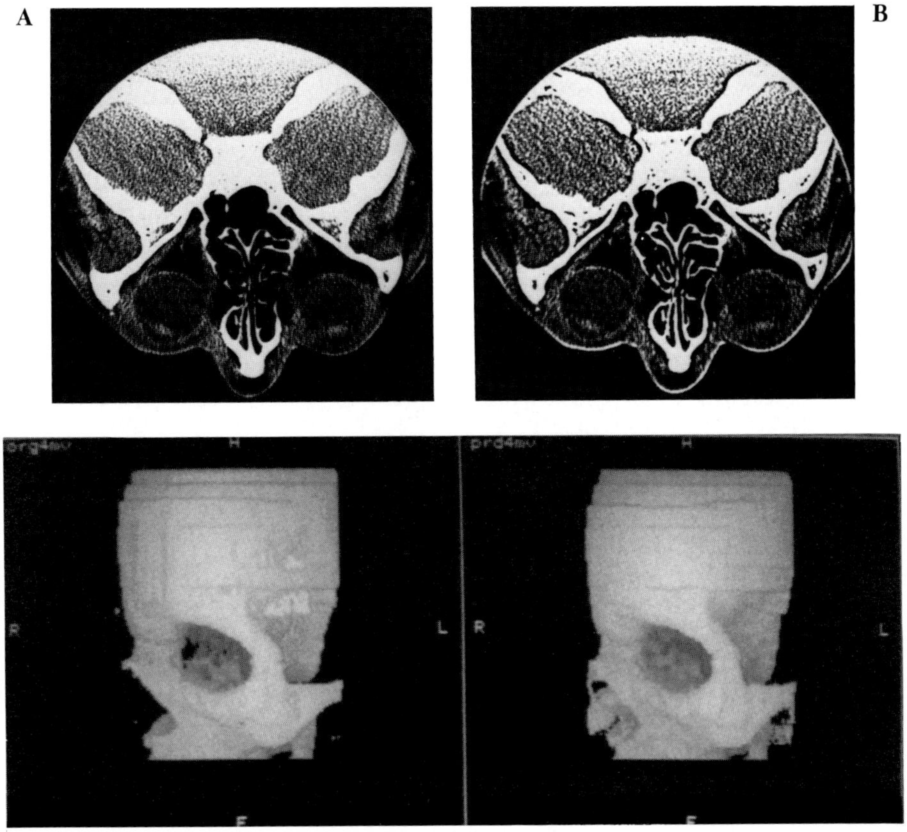

Fig. 2.7. Use of combined linear and nonlinear filtering to improve detection of papyraceous ethmoid bone. **A** Original CT slice. **B** Filtered CT slice. **C** Three-dimensional images before (left) and after (right) filtering to reduce "pseudo-foramina."

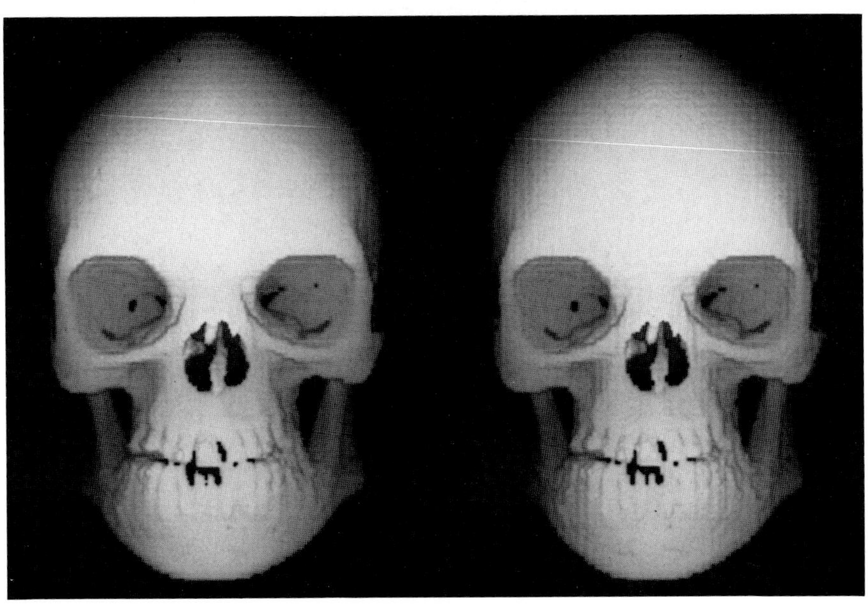

A

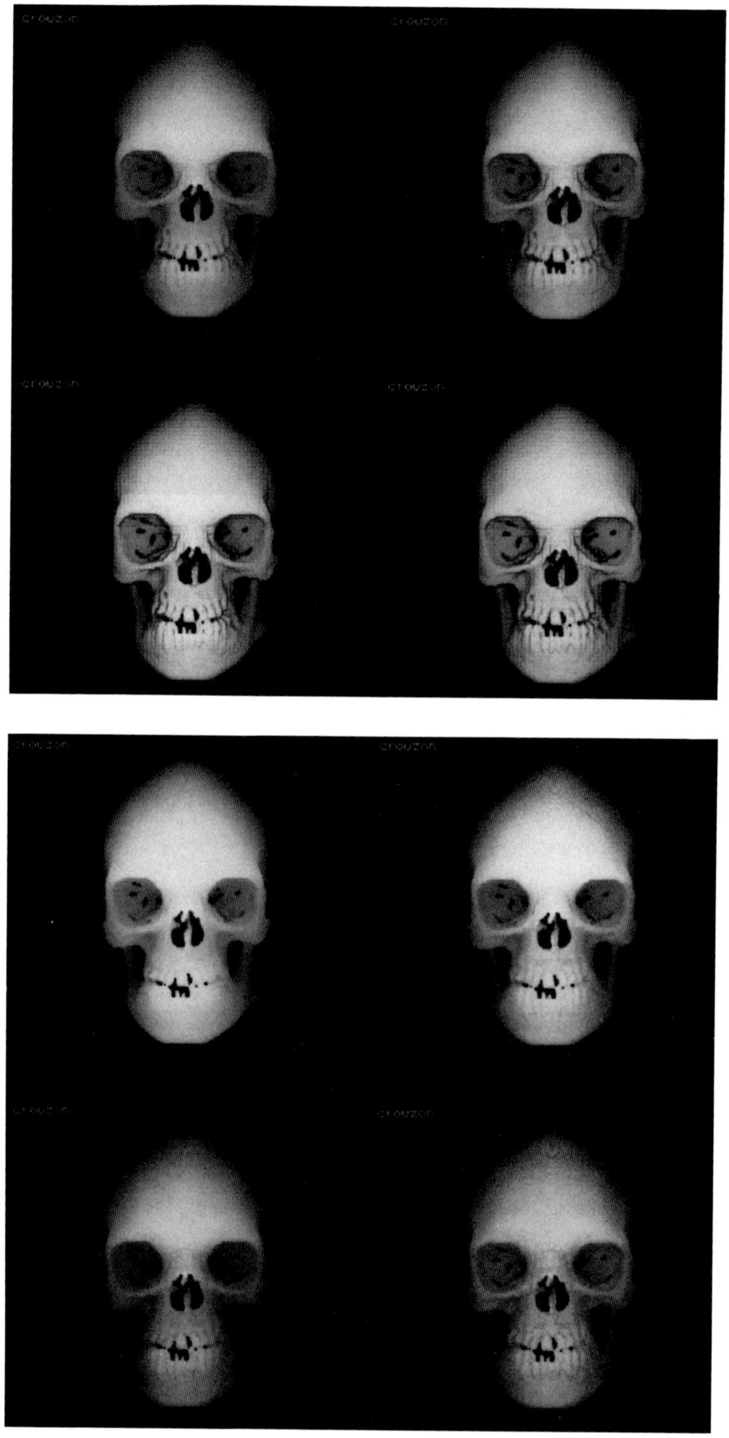

B

Fig. 2.9. **A** Gradient-based rendering. **B** Neighbor-based rendering.

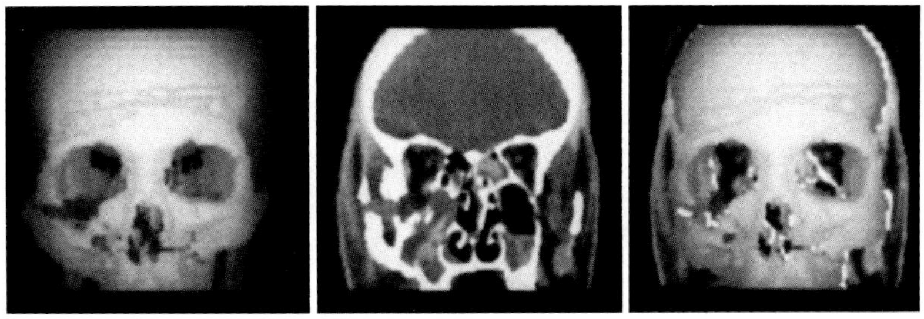

Fig. 2.10. Use of the 12-bit gray volume to display soft tissue along with bone.

A

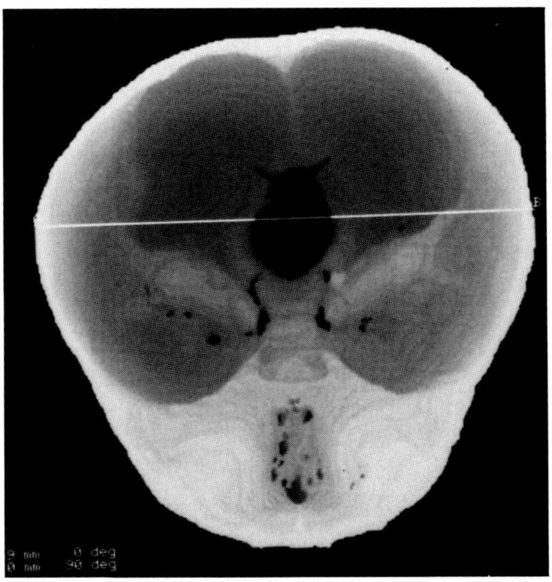

B

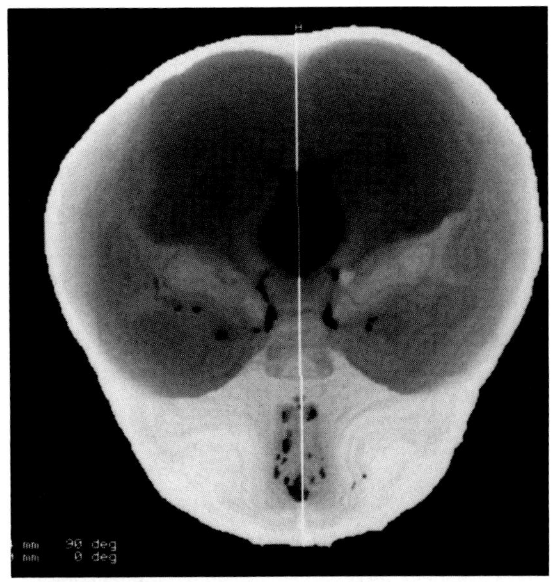

C

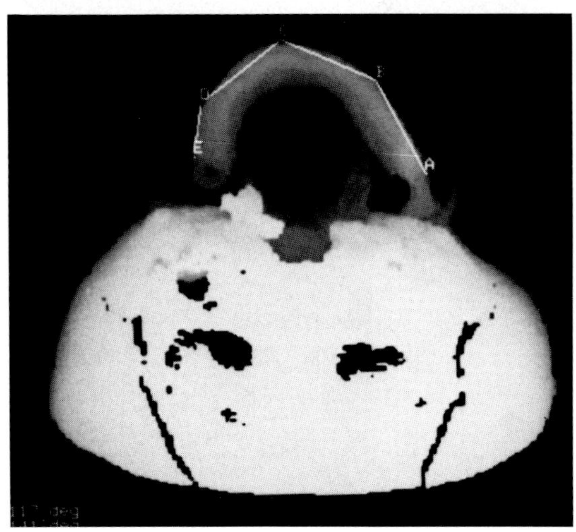

Fig. 2.11. Linear and angular measurements.

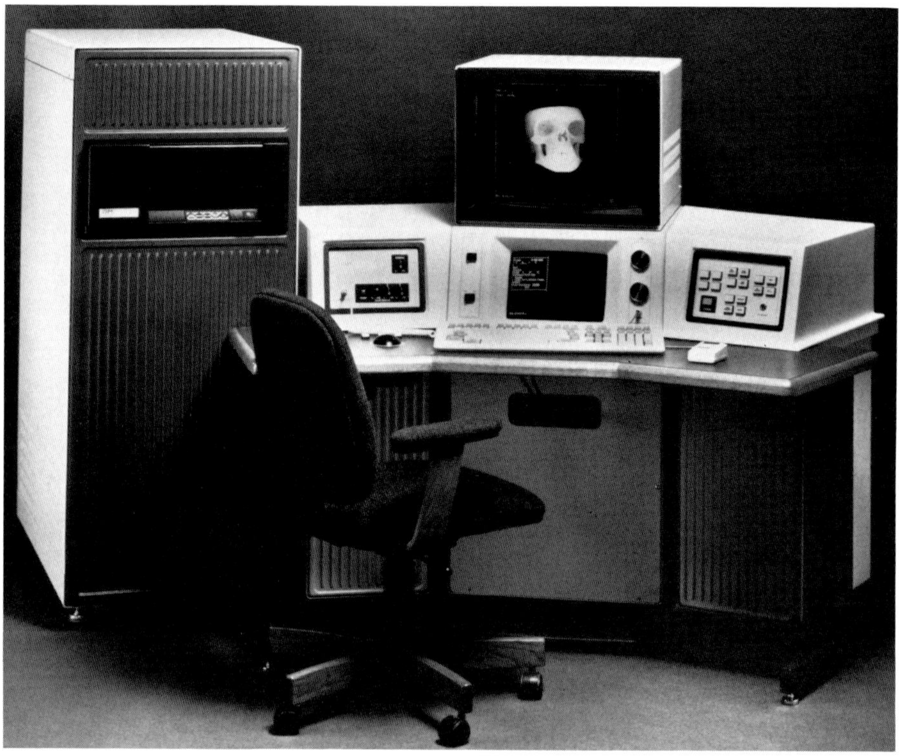

Fig. 2.12. Dedicated work station.

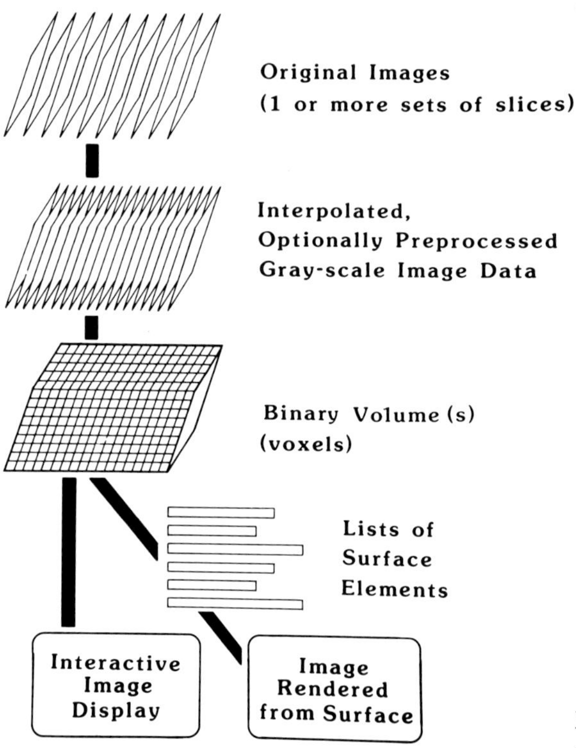

Fig. 2.13. Data flow in work station.

Fig. 2.16. Left: Image produced using laser imager. (Courtesy 3M Company.) Right: Image produced using standard multiformat camera. ▶

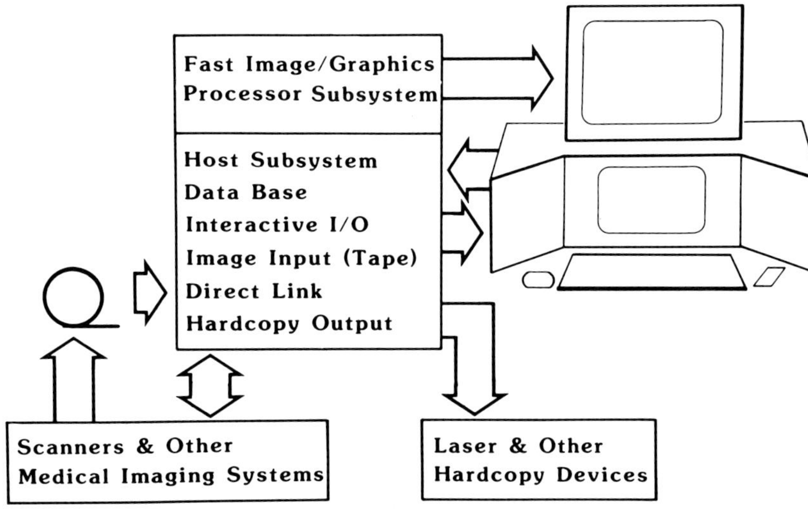

Fig. 2.14. Work station hardware components.

Fig. 2.15. Work station software components.

FOREGROUND (Interactive):	BACKGROUND:
Data Management	Data Input & Conversion
3-D Preparation	Batch MPR Computation
Interactive 3-D/MPR	Volume Computation
Image Review	Surface Computation
Snapshot Review	Batch Rendering

PRIMITIVES:	
Imaging	Interactive devices
Graphics	Menus
Data Base	

Unix Operating System
Custom Microcode
Device Drivers

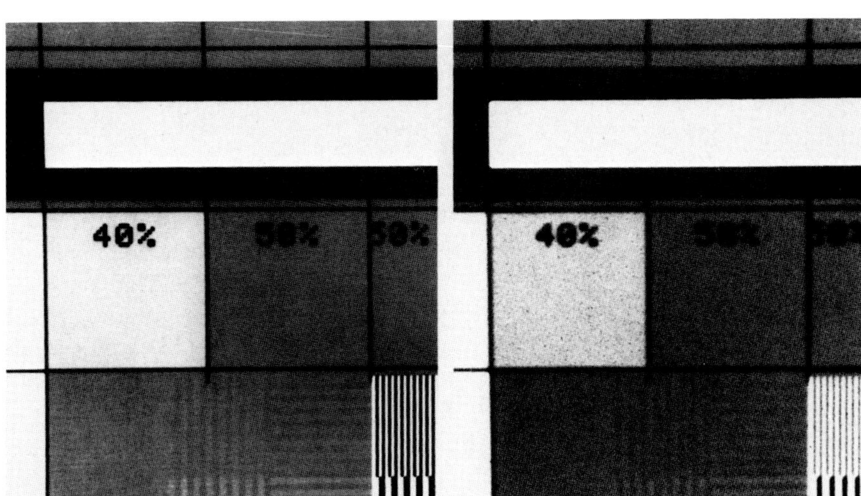

3

Normal Skull

Thresholding (*segmentation*), or the ability to distinguish one tissue from another, is affected by the relative difference in CT attenuation coefficients (CT numbers) of adjacent tissues or the thickness of the tissue of interest. A tissue contained in a heterogeneous medium, as occurs in vivo, is surrounded by other tissues of varying CT numbers. Differing tissues with CT numbers that approximate one another may offer indistinct margins for the application of segmentation techniques. This situation permits some modest variance from the real margins of the tissue. To demonstrate the degree of correspondence between the three-dimensional reconstructed skull and an anatomical specimen, we have purposely scanned these skulls in a medium of air to allow the greatest disparity between the osseous skull and the surrounding medium, thereby permitting the sharpest definition of the scanned skull. Furthermore, this method permits, in the development of the three-dimensional image, reduction of the "holes," or "pseudoforamina," that are produced by exclusion of bone containing voxels through false CT numbers by partial volume averaging. Nonetheless, many of the problems inherent in in vivo scanning are also present using this method. Surfaces of bone that are thin enough to permit translucency are not well represented by three-dimensional reconstruction. If a threshold for voxels containing these objects uses large CT values, papyraceous bone may not be included as part of the rendered object. One can then see the appearance of pseudoforamina. Selection of a smaller threshold value permits the representation of thin bone (without the appearance of translucency) at the expense of closure of many normal small foramina (Hemmy and Tessier, 1985). With present technology, then, it is recognized that in some areas, such as the lacrimal bone and the orbital plate of the ethmoid bone, there are inaccuracies; where bone is not represented, it may actually be present. Conversely, in neonatal skulls, lowering the threshold level to include thin bone may cause the appearance of closed sutures when indeed they are actually open. If the viewer bears these pitfalls in mind, there is generally little confusion between the normal and the abnormal skull.

Technique

The skulls included in this chapter were scanned using a General Electric 9800 scanner (General Electric Medical Systems, New Berlin, Wisconsin) with the gantry parallel to the orbitomeatal line. The 1.5 mm abutting CT slices were obtained using scanning factors of 125 kilovolts, 170 milliamperes, and a 3-second scan time. Equivalent views of the skulls of a term fetus, child, and 14-year-old are presented for comparison purposes. It is generally necessary to provide views around the interaural and spinal axes at 30° increments to display all foramina and sutures in proper relief, as these anatomical details become more apparent with changes in depth and surface normal shading. Although not illustrated here, the location of cephalometric points generally requires two or more views to provide the appropriate visual cues for location. Here also, changes in shading and view direction allow more accurate definition of a feature.

Recommended Reading

Hemmy DC, Tessier PL: CT of dry skulls with craniofacial deformities: Accuracy of three-dimensional reconstruction. Radiology 157:113–116, 1985.

A

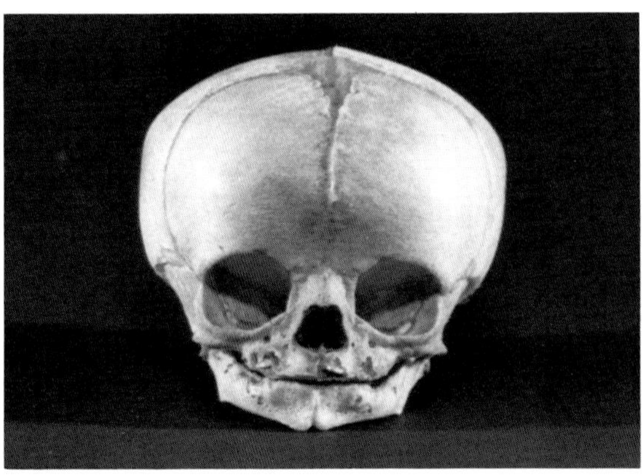

B

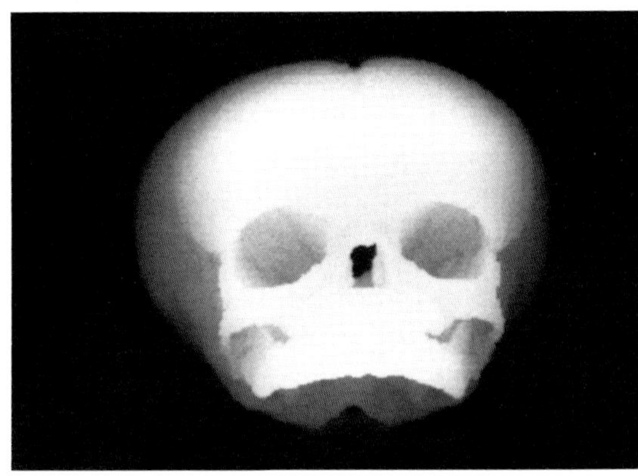

C

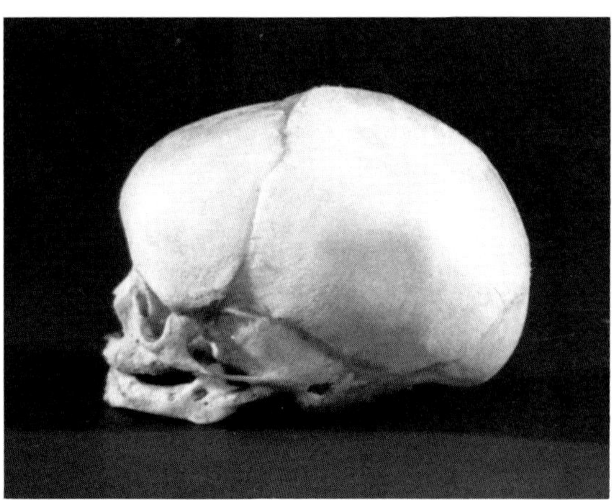

D

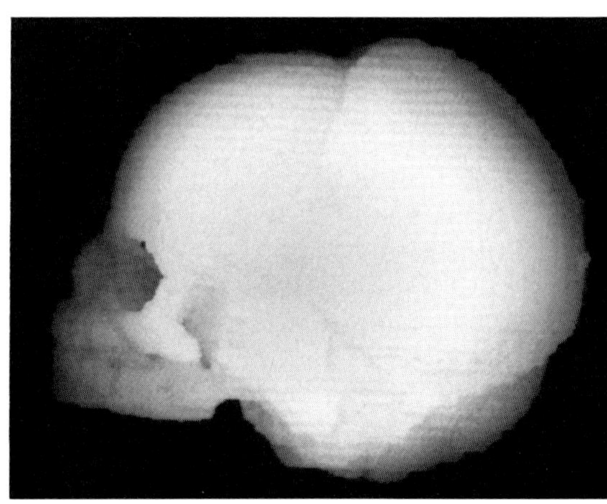

Fig. 3.1. Anterior and lateral views of skulls and three-dimensional reconstructions. **A,B,C,D** Fetus. **E,F,G,H** 7-Year-old child. **I,J,K,L** 14-Year-old child. Note the changes in craniofacial proportions and resultant morphology with advancing age. Note also the difficulty in accurately displaying the fetal skull due to thin bone. This does not occur in vivo.

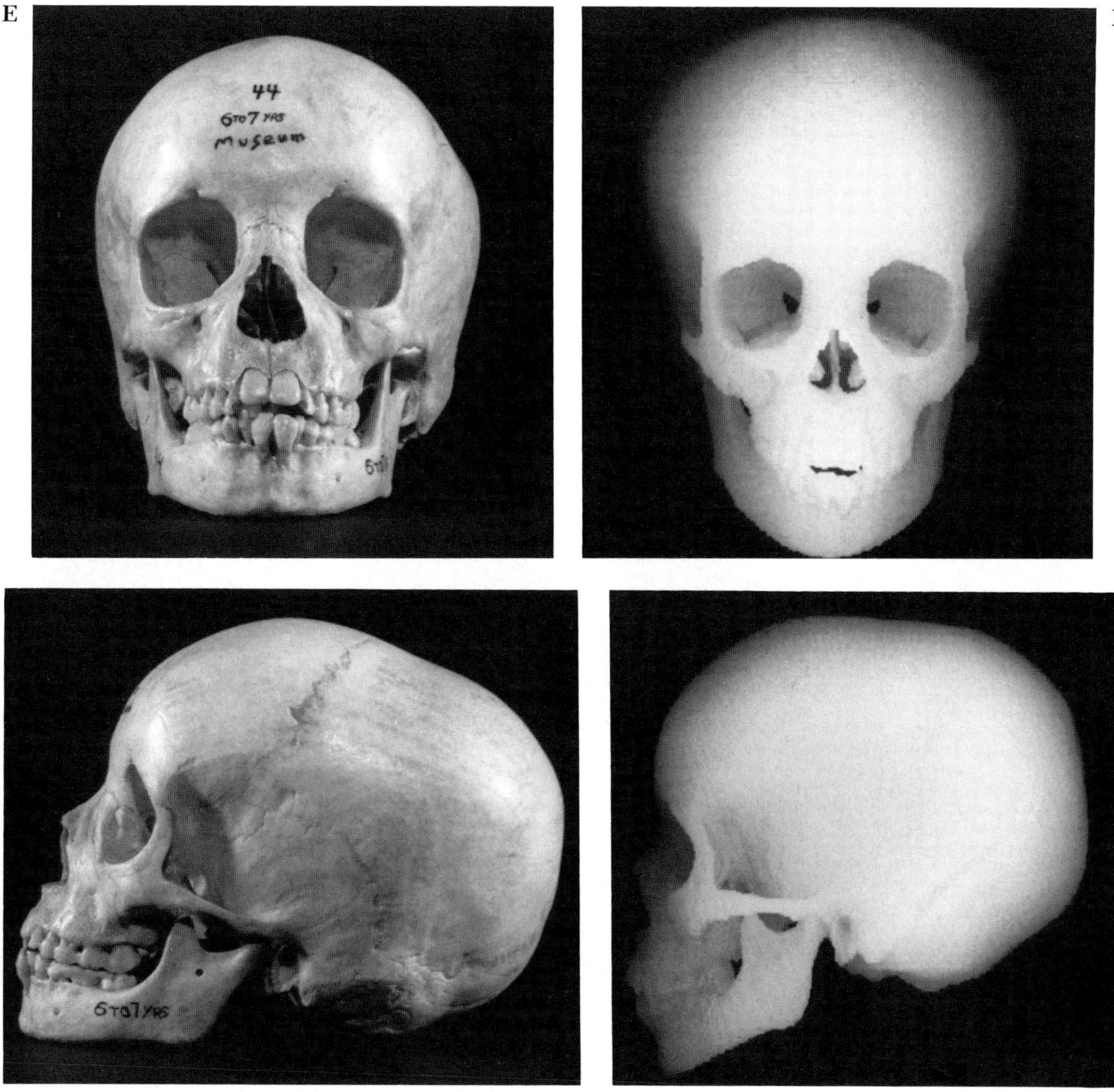

Fig. 3.1E–H. 7-year-old child.

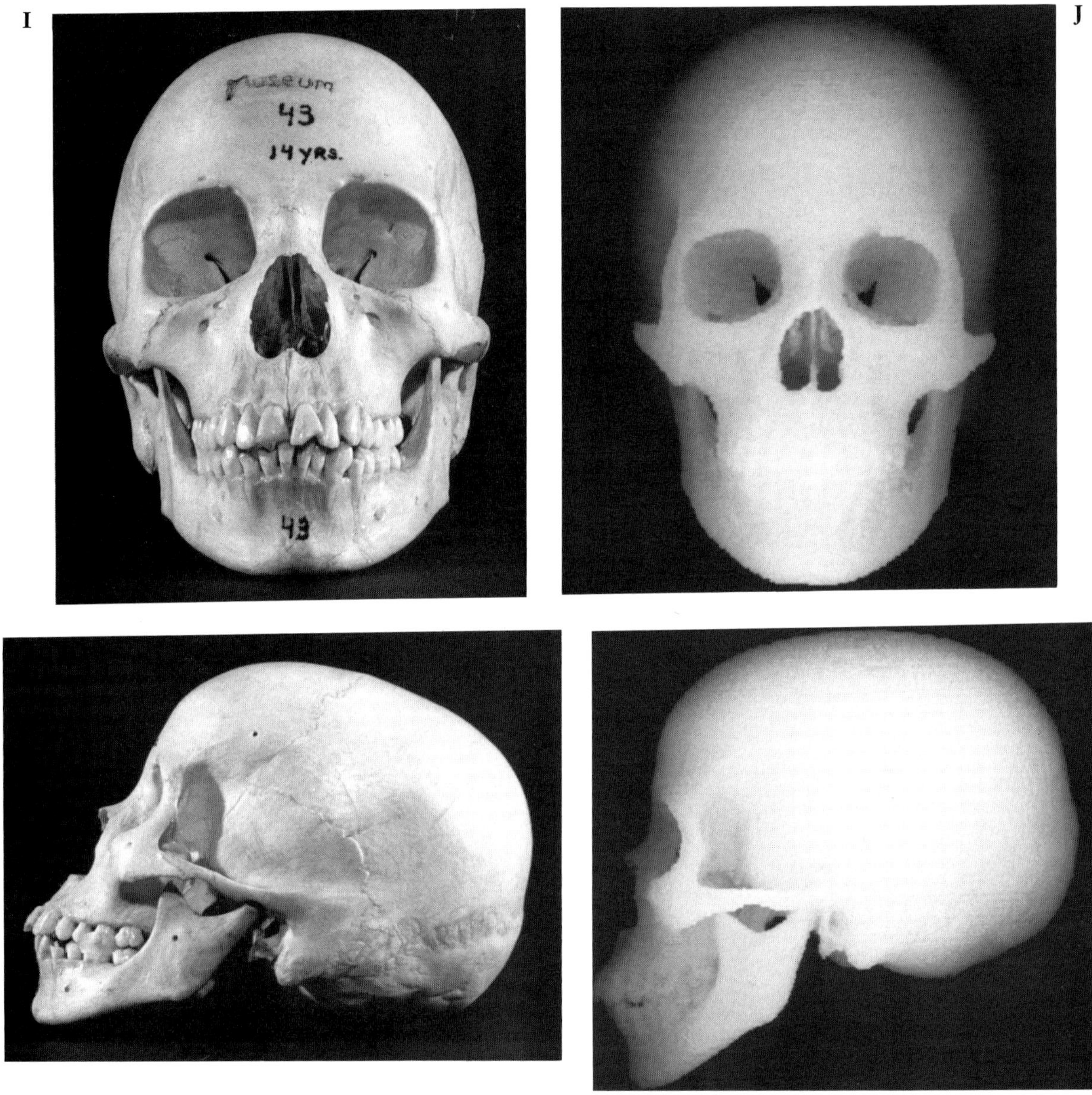

Fig. 3.1I–L. 14-year-old child.

A B C D E

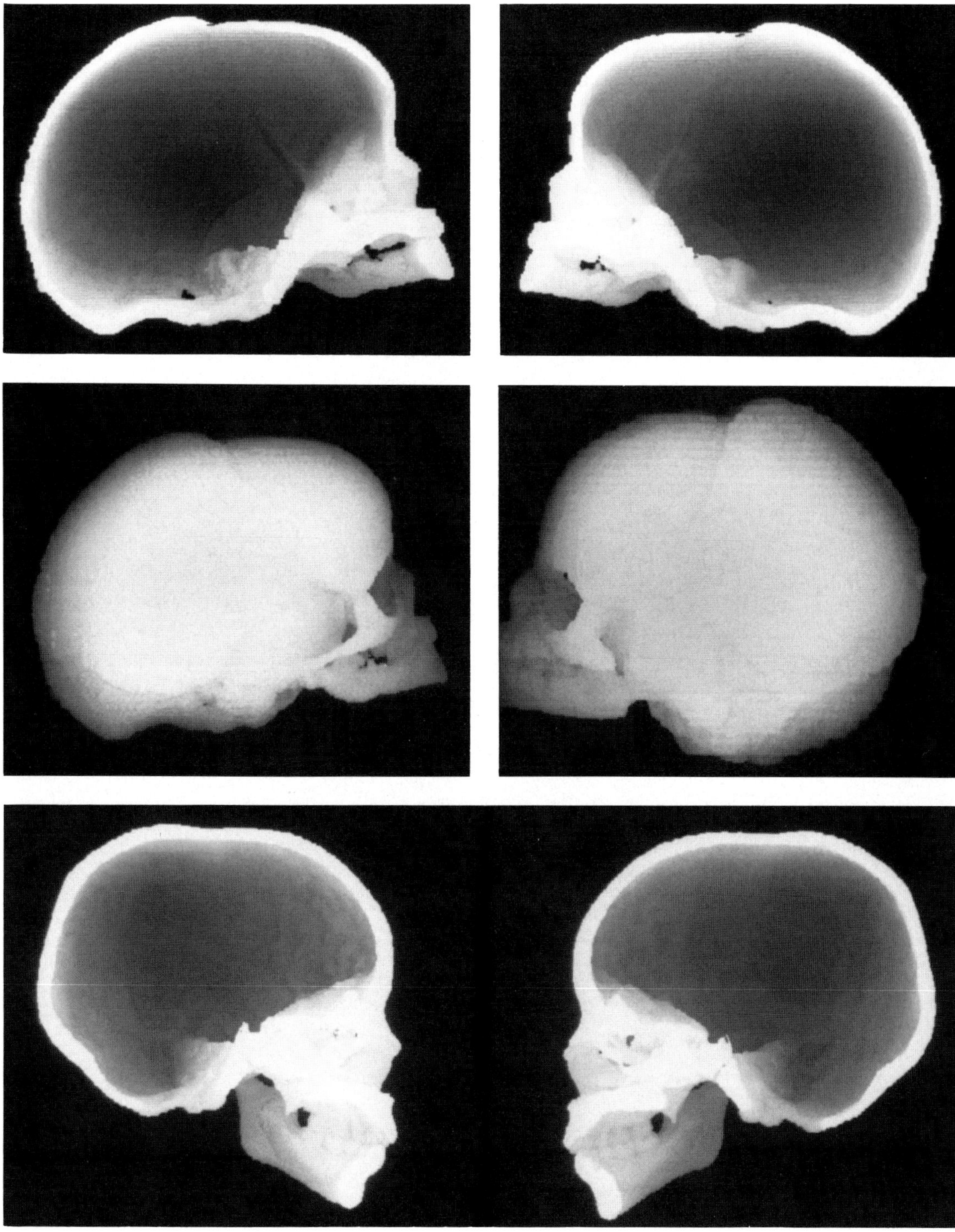

Fig. 3.2. Asymmetrical (2 mm off midline) display of the right and left halves of the skull. Observe the faithful display of sulcal impressions and vascular markings. Also note the representation of the vomer and relatively poor representation of the medial lamina of the ethmoid bone. Sphenooccipital synchrondrosis is well shown on the juvenile skull.

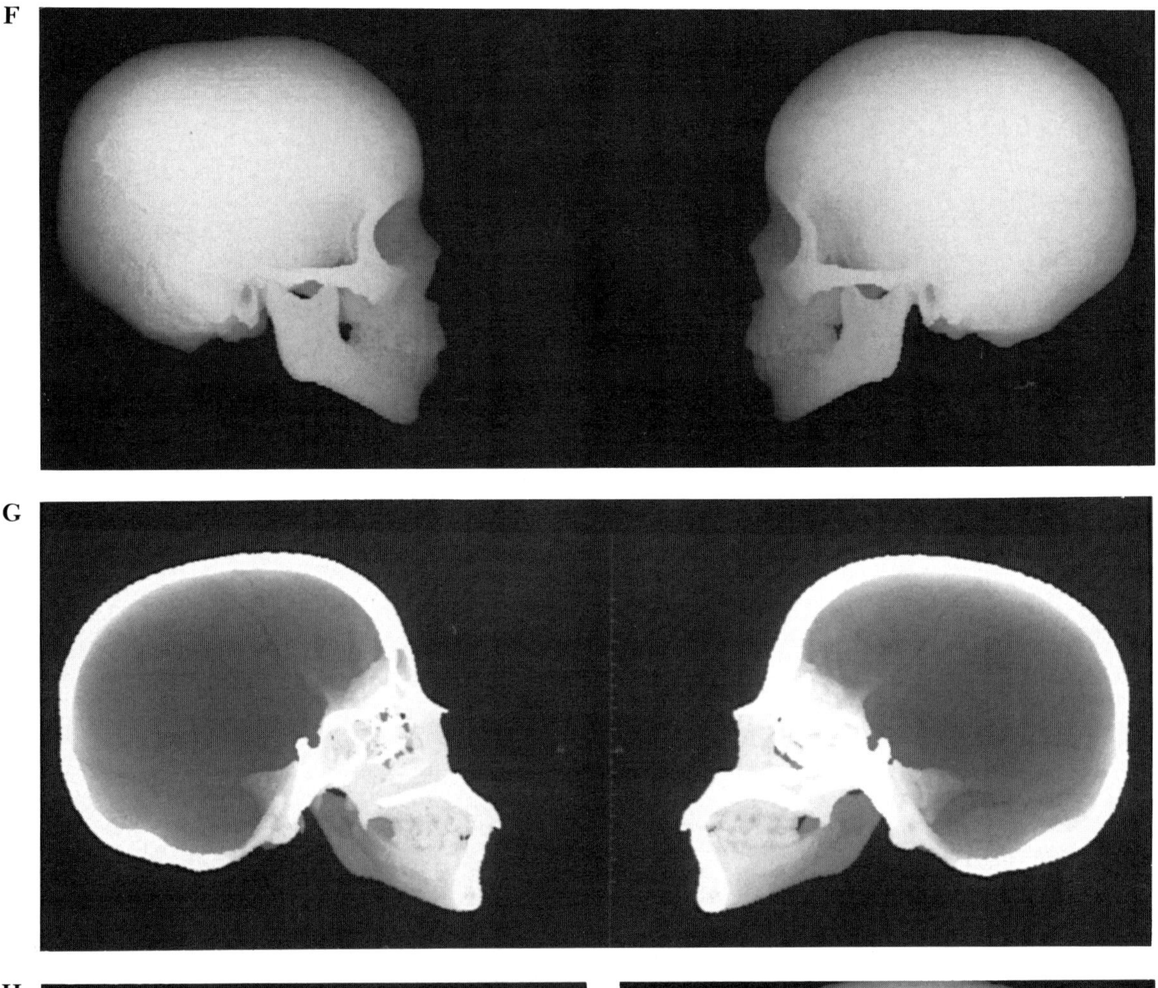

Fig. 3.2 (contd)

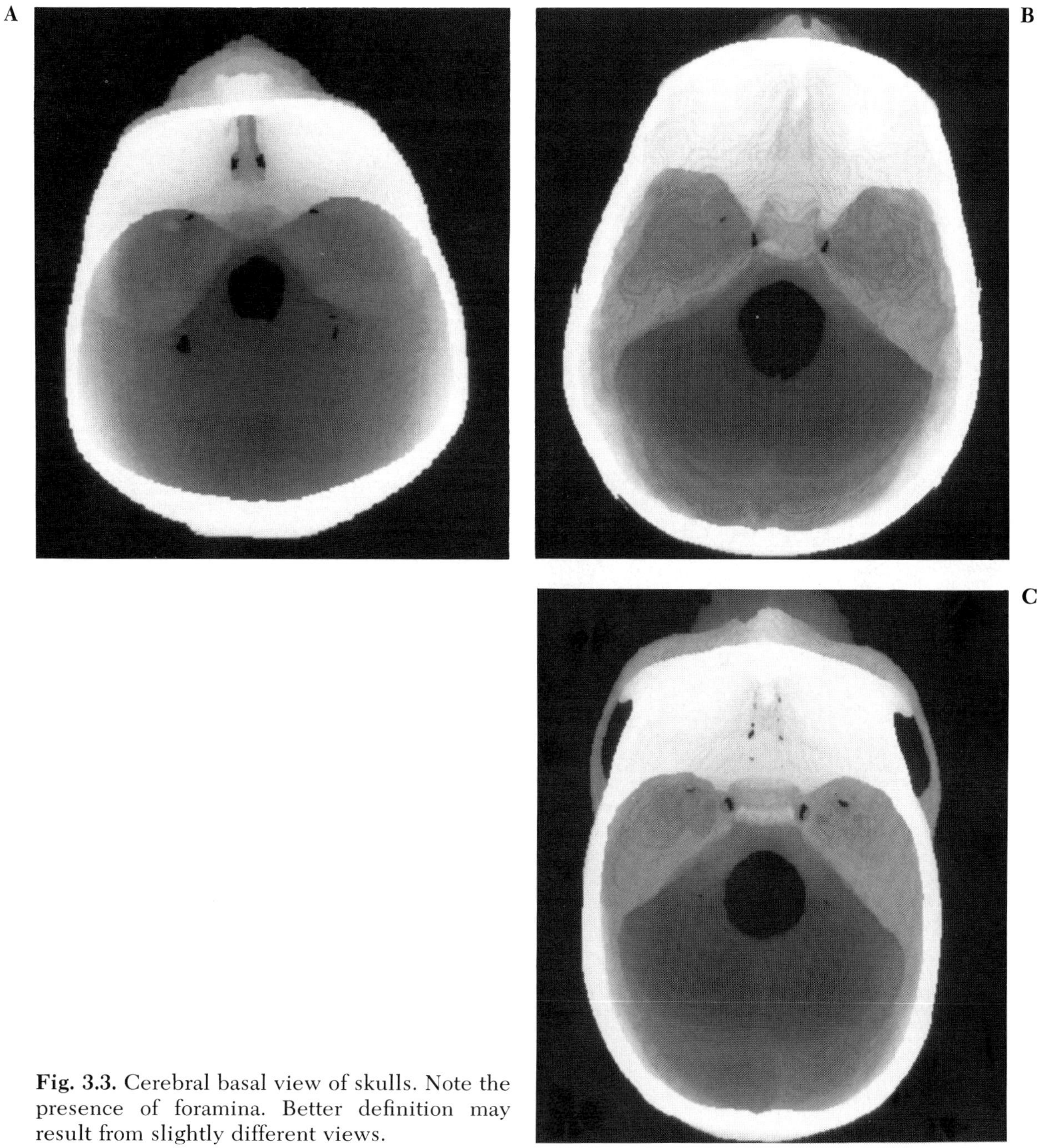

Fig. 3.3. Cerebral basal view of skulls. Note the presence of foramina. Better definition may result from slightly different views.

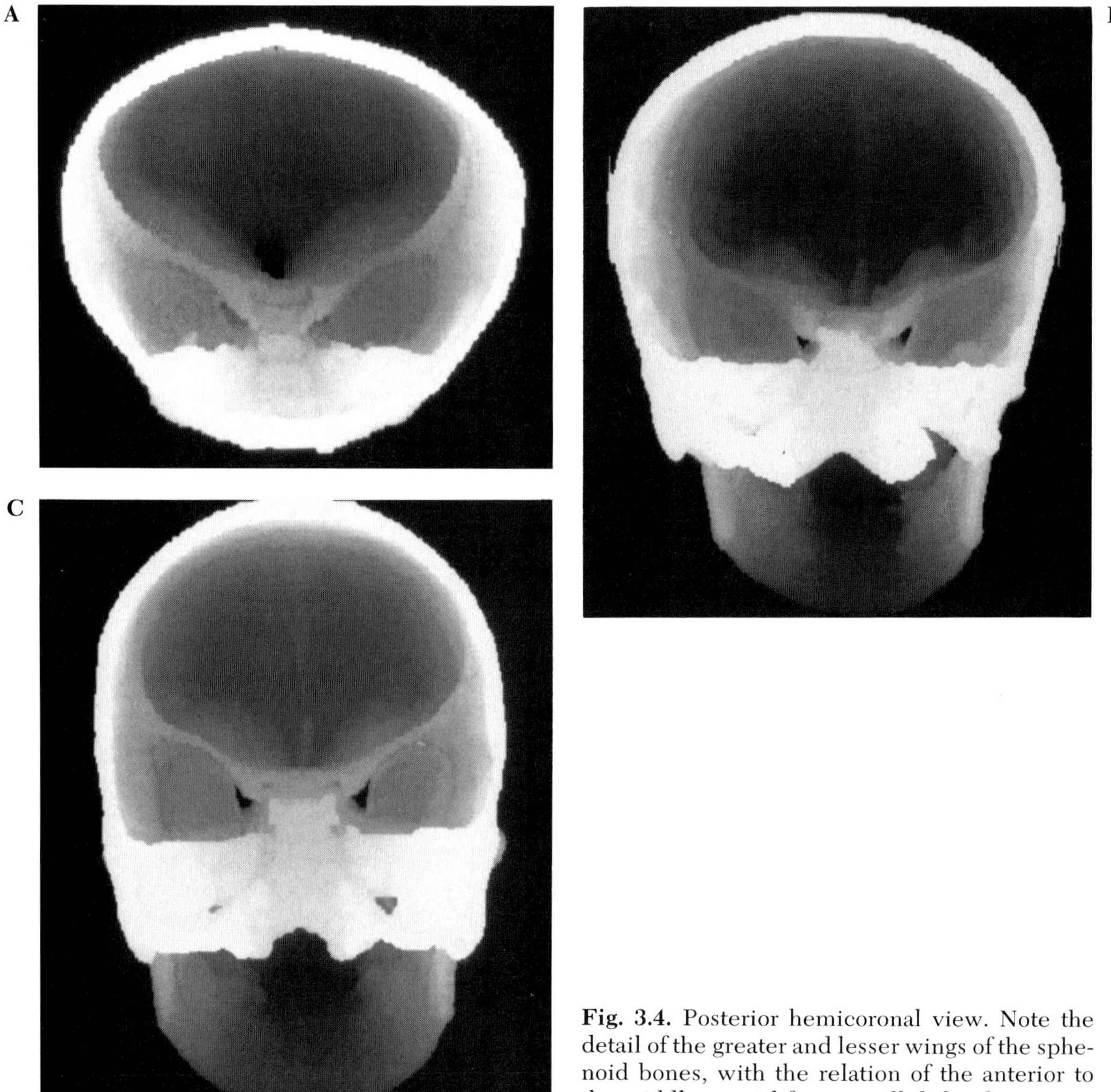

Fig. 3.4. Posterior hemicoronal view. Note the detail of the greater and lesser wings of the sphenoid bones, with the relation of the anterior to the middle cranial fossae well defined.

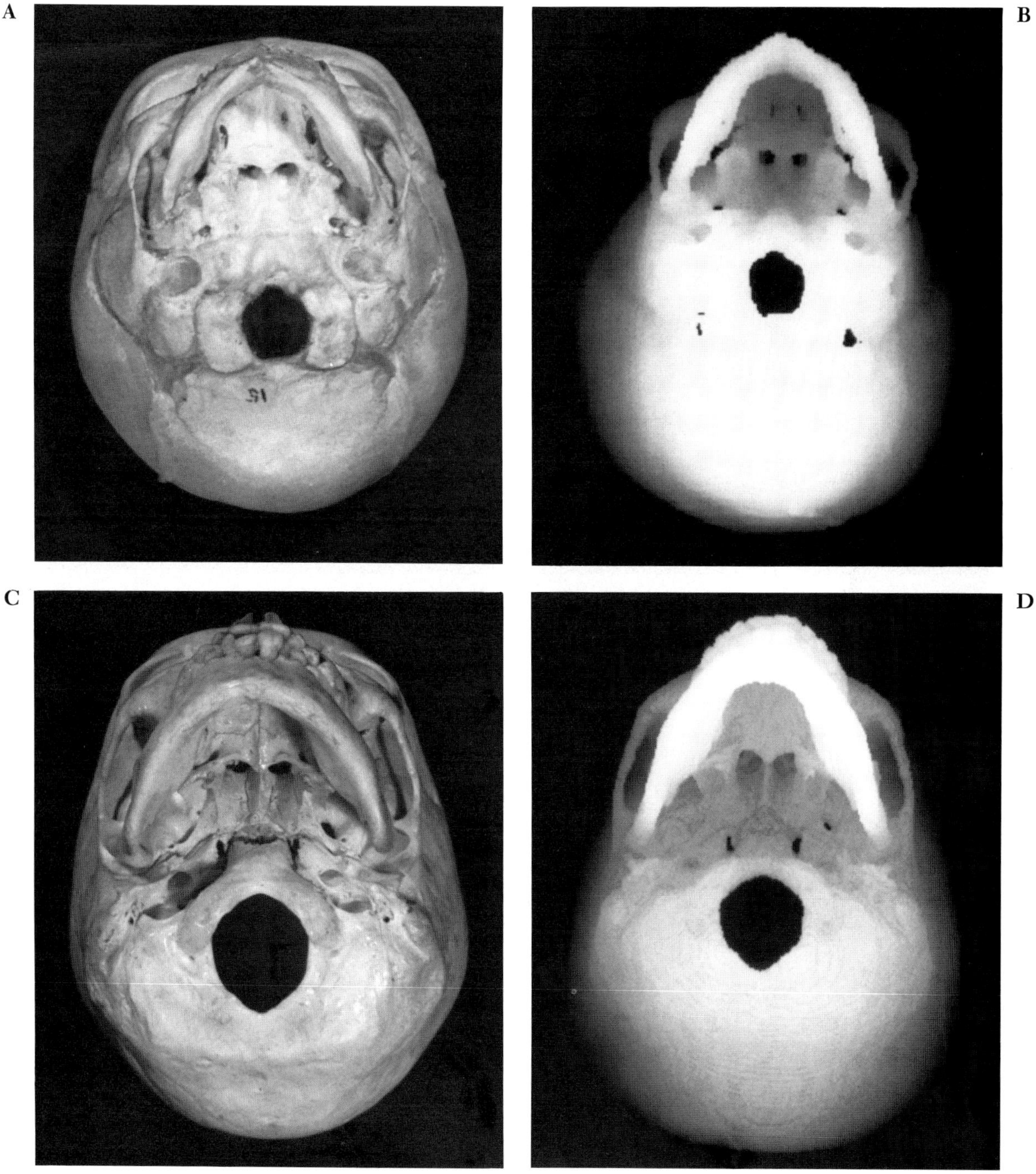

Fig. 3.5. Visceral basal view of skulls. Once again note the foraminal detail. Condylar emissary foramina can be easily seen.

E F

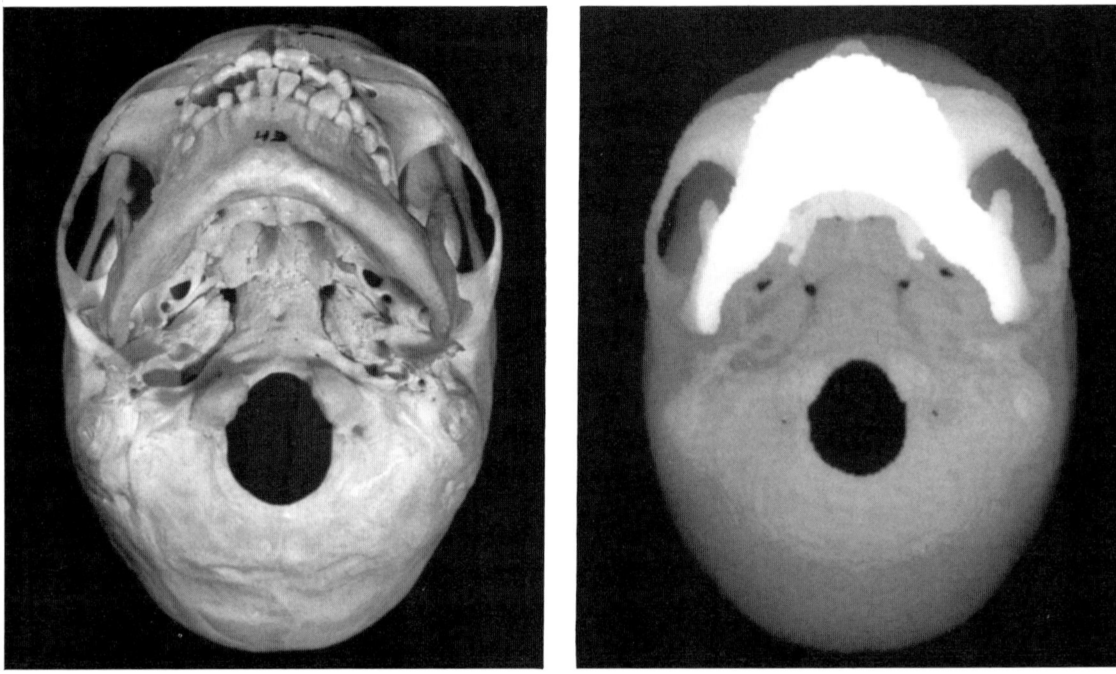

Fig. 3.5 (contd)

A

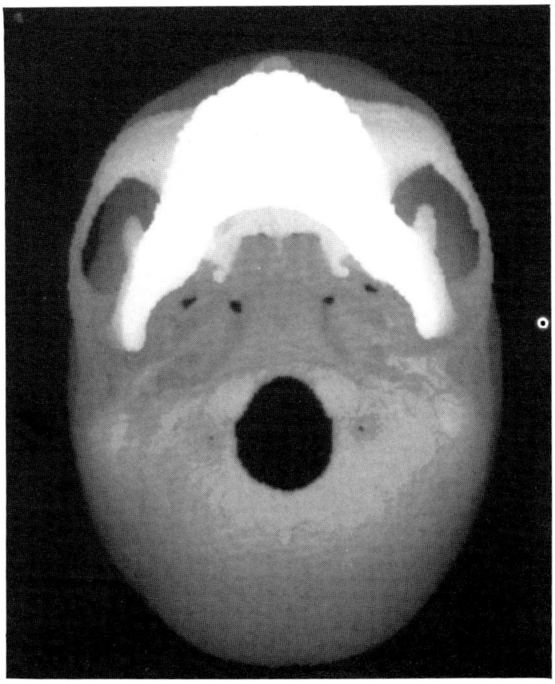

B

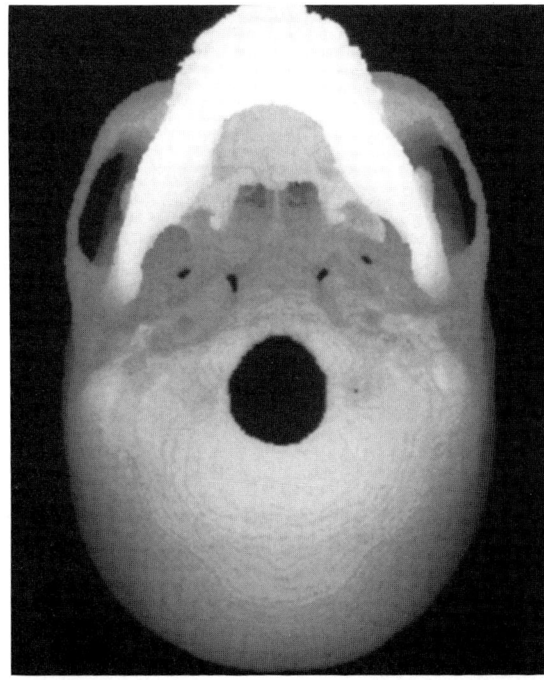

C

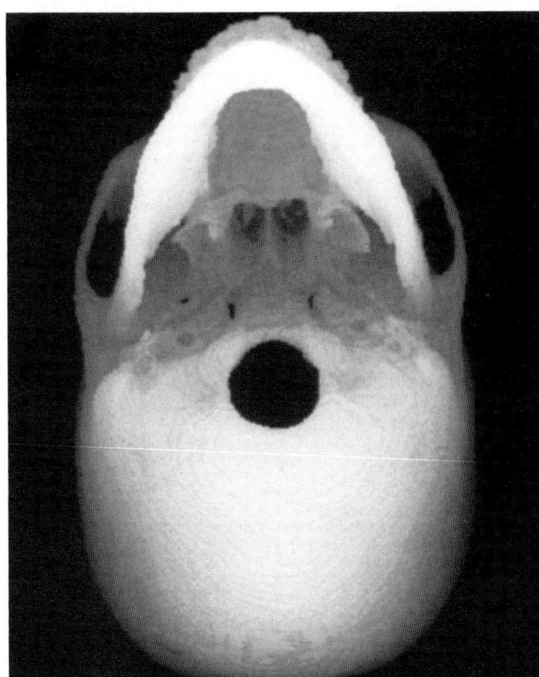

Fig. 3.6. Differing definition of skull with incremental rotation.

4

Craniosynostoses

The relation between skull deformities and premature fusion of the cranial sutures dates back to the beginning of the nineteenth century. Rudolph Virchow (1852) elaborated the concept and gave it wide currency, emphasizing that premature fusion of sutures was related to skull shape. With simple craniosynostosis there is premature fusion of one or more calvarial sutures without serious involvement of the facial skeleton or more convincing evidence that craniosynostosis is part of some recognizable malformation syndrome. However, in the more complex situations the abnormality is distributed throughout the skull. It is possible that the pathology starts in the cranial base; certainly in more complex deformities the skull base is involved, reflected in the calvaria above and the face below.

Three-dimensional imaging is now solidly contributing to our understanding of the disordered anatomy in these conditions. Studies that provide an examination of the cranial base and its neighboring structures demonstrate well the altered shapes of such bones as the sphenoid, which is considered to be the principal basal keystone. Using three-dimensional images the investigator is able to mentally assimilate a pattern of each deformity. Although individual sutures cannot yet be faithfully visualized by these techniques, it is the variation in shape, both symmetrical and asymmetrical, and the varying pattern of the craniosynostoses that are clearly depicted by three-dimensional imaging.

Craniosynostosis implies a change in volume of the cranial cavity and the orbits as well as in the volume of the naso-oropharynx. It is these volume changes that are of key clinical importance in craniostenosis, orbitostenosis, and faciostenosis. Three-dimensional imaging offers an exciting step toward objective volume measurement. Of importance to the interpretation of these images is a full appreciation of the two-dimensional CT data from which the final reconstructions are derived. Indeed, the value of the final three-dimensional images may be enhanced considerably by also referring to reformatted two-dimensional images.

Simple Calvarial Deformities

Scaphocephaly describes an abnormally long, narrow head (see Figs. 4.1 and 4.2). *Trigonocephaly* describes a head where the deformity consists of a narrow forehead with eyes that are usually closely set (see Fig. 4.3). *Turricephaly* describes an abnormally broad head with a high forehead. The highest point of the head may be anterior to the bregma (see Figs. 4.4 and 4.5). *Oxycephaly* refers to an abnormally high, conical head (see Fig. 4.6). *Plagiocephaly* is a term widely used to describe any lopsided, asymmetrical head (see Figs. 4.7 and 4.8). *Triphyllocephaly* is a term used to describe a trilobar head (see Figs. 4.9 and 4.10).

Scaphocephaly

Scaphocephaly is the most common of the calvarial deformities associated with craniosynostosis. The name "boat head" is apt: The skull is long and narrow, like a boat upside down (Figs. 4.1 and 4.2), and there is often a median ridge that simulates the keel (Fig. 4.2C). The forehead is usually high and prominent, with well developed frontal bosses (Fig. 4.1D); the skull slopes back to the occiput, which is prominent in profile (Fig. 4.2D) and often somewhat wedge-shaped as seen from the vertex view. This deformity is usually associated with premature closure of the anterior fontanelle and premature fusion of the sagittal suture (Fig. 4.2E). However, there are occasional patients with scaphocephaly who have premature fusion of other sutures, especially the coronal suture.

Trigonocephaly

Trigonocephaly is a wedge-shaped congenital deformity of the frontal region with a median bony ridge extending from the glabella to the bregmatic region (Fig. 4.3). The deformity is associated with premature fusion of the metopic suture. Normally the metopic suture is present at birth and does not begin to close until the second year of life.

Turricephaly

Turricephaly is characterized by an abnormally tall, broad head (Figs. 4.4 and 4.5). In profile, the front of the head looks high and slopes back to the occiput, which is less prominent than usual. The vertex of the head is often rather far forward, at or near the bregma (Fig. 4.4E). The forehead is steep and high, often broad, and usually rather flattened; there is a relative recession of the glabella (Figs. 4.4C,E). There may be mild hypertelorism. The lower face is usually unremarkable (Figs. 4.4A,B,D and 4.5A,B). Characteristically, both coronal sutures are fused (Fig. 4.5E), although other sutures may be involved.

Oxycephaly

With oxycephaly (Fig. 4.6), the head is more pointed (Fig. 4.6A–C), and fusion of the sagittal suture is more conspicuous. However, the deformity is similar to turricephaly, and some clinicians do not try to distinguish them.

Plagiocephaly

Plagiocephaly, a common deformity, is characterized by cranial and facial asymmetry (Figs. 4.7 and 4.8). The asymmetries can be complex and difficult to classify. The orbits may be asymmetrical in shape and in relation to each other, in both horizontal and vertical planes (Figs. 4.7B,C and 4.8C,E), resulting in hypertelorism and orbital dystopia, respectively. The face also shows three-dimensional asymmetry, and there is often a curvature in relation to the vertical axis (facial scoliosis). However, fairly consistent clinical patterns of plagiocephaly can be recognized. There are three defined subgroups.

Frontal plagiocephaly corresponds with unicoronal synostosis (Fig. 4.7). It forms the largest group of plagiocephalic craniosynostoses and may be an important cause of cosmetic disability.

Occipital plagiocephaly may be associated with lambdoid synostosis or, at least, with intrinsic cranial growth delay in the lambdoid zone.

Parallelogram plagiocephaly has been defined as expressing severe unilateral cranial growth delay, with premature fusion of the coronal, squamosal, and lambdoid sutures in various combinations. It is a noticeable deformity (Fig. 4.8).

Craniofacial Syndromes

Craniofacial syndromes are the forms of craniosynostosis in which abnormal calvarial growth is associated with disturbances of facial growth of equal or greater importance. Cohen (1979) has listed 57 syndromes associated with craniosynostosis, and his summaries indicate that most of these syndromes include abnormal facies among their manifestations. Consideration is given here only to those syndromes that are reasonably common and that are known to present important clinical challenges.

Crouzon Syndrome

Crouzon syndrome is the most common craniofacial syndrome. It was first described in 1912 by Crouzon, who clearly recognized the triad of calvarial deformity, facial deformity, and exophthalmos (Figs. 4.9 and 4.10). The skull deformities are invariably associated with extensive premature fusion of calvarial sutures, but the craniosynostosis is never confined to a single suture or sutural system. In most cases, all calvarial sutures eventually undergo premature fusion, and the basal sutures may fuse prematurely as well. Other abnormalities in the skull base include hypoplasia of the entire anterior fossa and a deep sella turcica. Orbitostenosis may be extreme, with resultant exophthalmos and visual axes that tend to diverge (Figs. 4.9J,N,O). Maxillary hypoplasia is a cardinal part of the syndrome and determines the characteristic appearance of the middle face (Figs. 4.10D,E and 4.11B): The cheeks are flat, the upper lip is inconspicuous, and the lower jaw is relatively prognathous (Figs. 4.10A–C and 4.11A,C). The nose, being less affected by the failure of growth in membranous bones, stands out prominently. The faciostenosis of Crouzon syndrome constricts the nasal air passages, and there may be posterior choanal atresia. The shortening of the maxilla places the upper incisors well behind the mandibular incisors, and the narrowing of the maxilla compounds the malocclusion by causing bilateral crossbite and crowding of teeth (Figs. 4.11B,D). The palate is high and narrow, and this deformity is accentuated during childhood, with increasing disproportion between the normal growth of the teeth and abnormal growth of the maxilla. The faciostenosis also distorts speech. Patients often develop increased intracranial pressure as a consequence of craniostenosis (Figs. 4.9I,M and 4.10E,F). It is generally agreed that Crouzon syndrome is inherited as a mendelian dominant gene of high penetrance (Figs. 4.9A–G).

Apert Syndrome

Apert syndrome is the second most common craniofacial syndrome. It was first described in 1906 by Apert, who termed the condition acrocephalosyndactyly. The cranial deformity is almost always associated with premature fusion of the coronal sutures, although the skull base is also involved. Apert syndrome is distinguished from other acrocephalosyndactylies by the severity of the syndactyly. The head is usually turricephalic with a high forehead and flattened occiput (Figs. 4.12, 4.13, 4.14, and 4.15). At birth, the anterior fontanelle and the metopic suture are usually wide open and may remain so for some months (Figs. 4.12D,E and 4.13C–F). There is upward slanting obliquity of the orbital roof, so characteristic of turricephaly, and there may be true orbital hypertelorism (Figs. 4.12C,E, 4.13C–F, and 4.14C). The facial deformities are striking: The maxilla is hypoplastic (Figs. 4.12D,E, 4.13A–F, and 4.15E), the nose and lower jaw are relatively prominent, and the eyes are wide apart. The face is frequently asymmetrical: The nose may deviate, and there is often a frontal plagiocephaly. The palatal arch is high and narrow, an appearance exaggerated by hypertrophy along the alveolar margins. The upper teeth are crowded together (Fig. 4.15C), and there is usually a class III malocclusion with an open bite (Fig. 4.15E). These deformities combine to affect speech and are often compounded by intellectual retardation. Syndactyly of hands and feet is a universal and specific component of the syndrome, with the hands being spoon-shaped and with fusion of at least the middle three digits. The toes are affected in a similar way. Apert syndrome appears to be related to increased paternal age; and although most cases are sporadic, it is an autosomal dominant trait.

Saethre-Chotzen Syndrome

Saethre-Chotzen syndrome, one of the commoner complex craniofacial syndromes, was apparently first reported in 1931 by Saethre of Oslo. The skull is usually brachycephalic, and often plagiocephaly is present with partial or complete premature coronal synostosis (Fig. 4.16). The craniosynostosis seen with this syndrome may be comparatively minor, but the facial appearance can be distressing. The facial asymmetry is often aggravated by hypertelorism and orbital dystopia (Fig. 4.16A,B). The frontal hairline is low, and mild ptosis is often evident. The nose may be beaked with septal deviation, and the maxillary complex is often hypoplastic. When present, the syndactyly may be mild with only webbing of the second and third digits in the hands and feet. Saethre-Chotzen syndrome usually shows autosomal dominant inheritance with high penetrance and variable expression.

Cohen Syndrome

Cohen described in 1979 a form of frontonasal dysplasia that produces craniosynostosis and is inherited as a dominant trait. Although rare, these patients have brachycephaly with premature coronal synostosis, bilateral or unilateral (Fig. 4.17). The facial deformities are characteristic with extreme ocular and orbital hypertelorism with wide telecanthus (Fig. 4.17A,B). The nose is broad with a bifid tip. Most recorded cases include minor abnormalities in the digits, long bones, or both, with mild syndactyly being most common.

Pfeiffer Syndrome

The constellation of craniosynostosis, widening of the thumbs and great toes, and partial syndactyly of the fingers is characteristic of Pfeiffer syndrome (Fig. 4.18). This disorder, first reported in 1964, has autosomal dominant inheritance. The craniosynostosis is associated with maxillary hypoplasia (Figs. 4.18C,D), orbital proptosis (Figs. 4.18A,B), and hypertelorism (Figs. 4.18A–E).

Recommended Reading

Apert E: De l'acrocéphalosyndactylie. Bull Soc Med Paris 23:1310, 1906.

Cohen MM Jr: Craniosynostosis and syndromes with craniosynostosis: incidence, genetics, penetrance, variability and new syndrome updating. Birth Defects 15(5B):13, 1979.

Cohen MM Jr (ed): Craniosynostosis. Diagnosis, Evaluation and Management. Raven Press, New York, 1986.

Crouzon O: Dysostose cranio-faciale héréditaire. Bull Soc Med Hop Paris 33:545, 1912.

David DJ, Poswillo D, Simpson D: The Craniosynostoses. Causes, Natural History, and Management. Springer-Verlag, New York, 1982.

Dufresne CR, McCarthy JG, Cutting CB, et al: Volumetric quantification of intracranial and ventricular volume following cranial vault remodeling: a preliminary report. Plast Reconstr Surg 79:24, 1987.

Ingraham FD, Matson DD: Neurosurgery of Infancy and Childhood. Charles C Thomas, Springfield, Ill, 1954.

Kreiborg S: Crouzon syndrome: a clinical and roentgen-cephalometric study. Scand J Plast Reconstr Surg, suppl 18, 1981.

Marchac D, Renier D: Craniofacial Surgery for Craniosynostosis. Little, Brown, Boston, 1982.

Montaut J, Stricker M: Les dysmorphies craniofaciales—les synostoses prématurées (craniosténoses et faciosténoses). Neurochirurgie 23, suppl 2, 1977.

Pfeiffer RA: Dominant erbliche Akrocephalosyndaktylie. Z Kinderheilkd 90:301, 1964.

Saethre H: Ein Beitrag zum Turmschädelproblem (Pathogenese, Erblichkeit und Symptomatologie). Z Nervenheilkd 117:533, 1931.

Tessier P: Relationship of craniostenosis to craniofacial dysostoses, and to faciostenoses: a study with therapeutic implications. Plast Reconstr Surg 48:224, 1971.

Tessier P: Recent improvements in treatment of facial and cranial deformities of Crouzon's disease and Apert's syndrome. In Tessier P, Callahan A, Mustarde JC, Salyer K (eds): Symposium on Plastic Surgery in the Orbital Region (Proceedings, Symposium of the Educational Foundation of the American Society of Plastic and Reconstructive Surgery, (vol. 12). Mosby, St. Louis, p 271, 1976.

Virchow R: Über den Cretinismus, namentlich in Franken, und über pathologische Schädelformen. Verh Phys Med Ges Würzburg 2:230, 1851–1852.

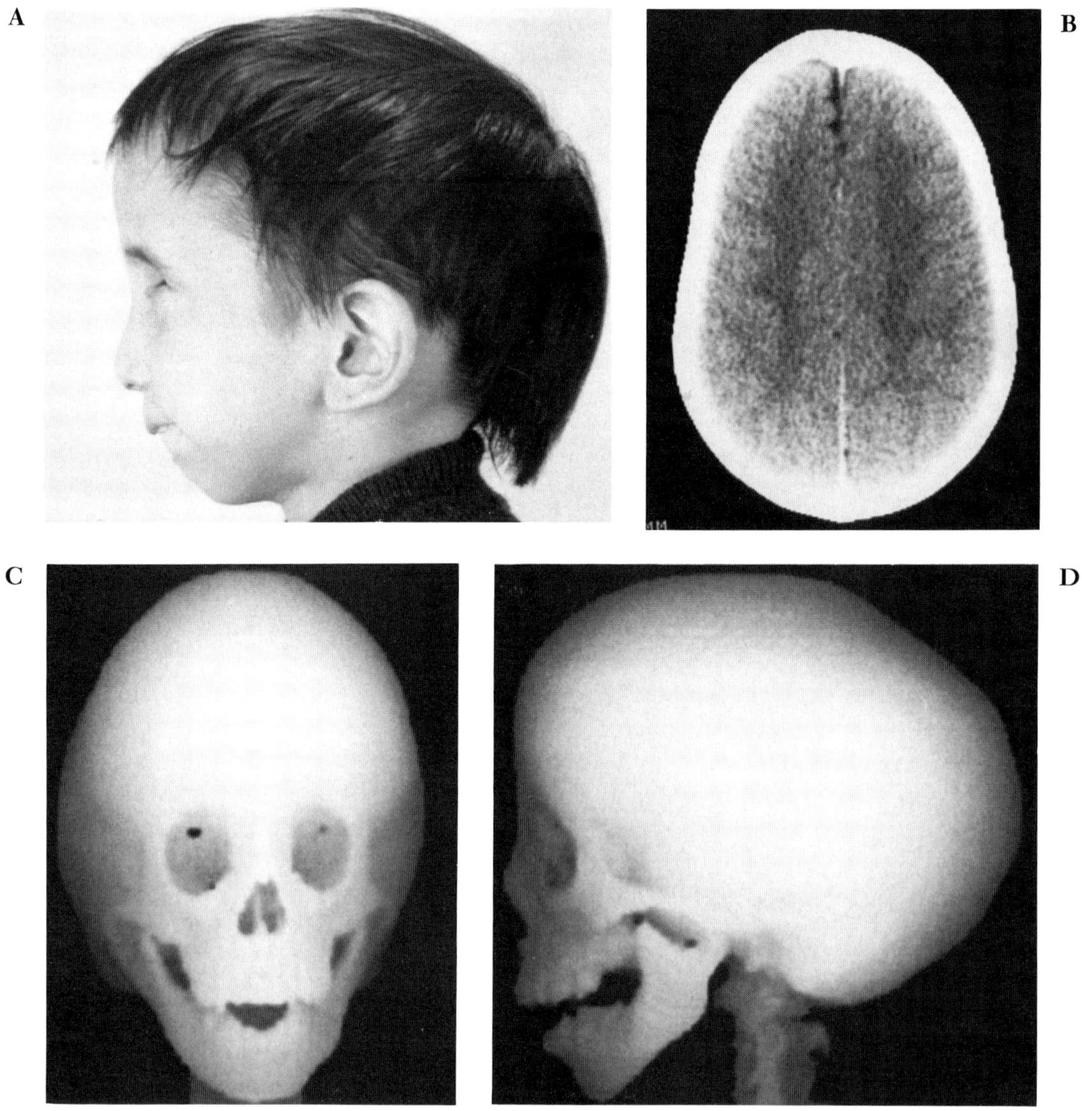

Fig. 4.1. **A** Scaphocephalic head is long and has a high, prominent forehead. **B** Axial CT slice shows the long, narrow head surrounding normal brain. **C** There may be hypotelorism. **D** Frontal and occipital prominences make significant contributions to skull length.

A B C D

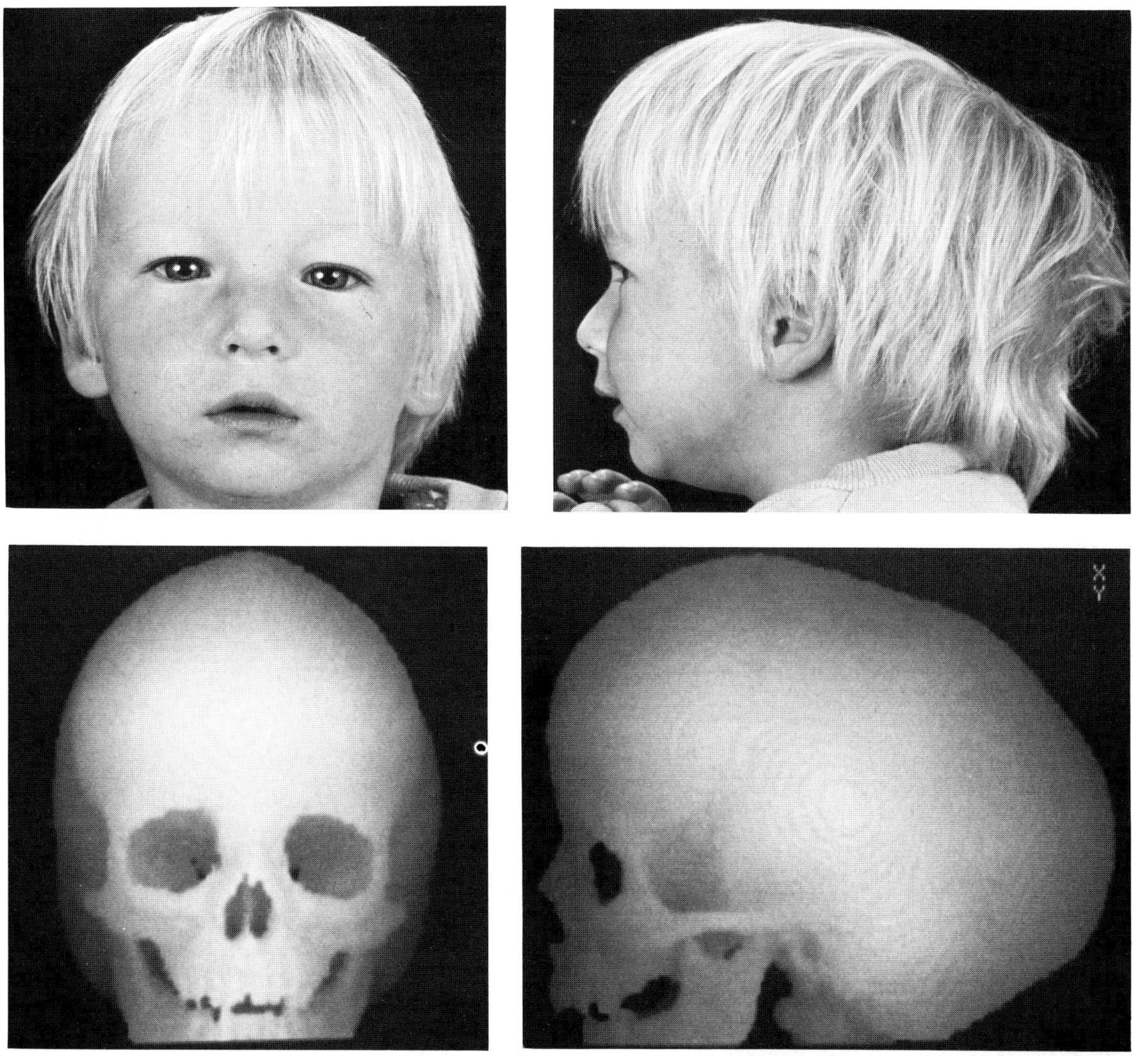

E

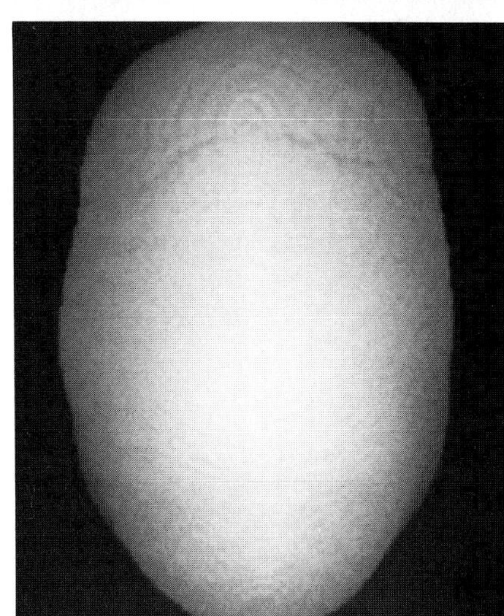

Fig. 4.2. **A** Forehead sweeps up to a median ridge. **B** Scaphocephalic head shape is best appreciated in the lateral view. **C** "Keel-like" deformity at the vertex results from premature sagittal sutural fusion. **D** Frontal and occipital bossing. **E** In a view from the vertex, the coronal sutures can be seen anteriorly, but there is no sign of the sagittal suture.

A B C D

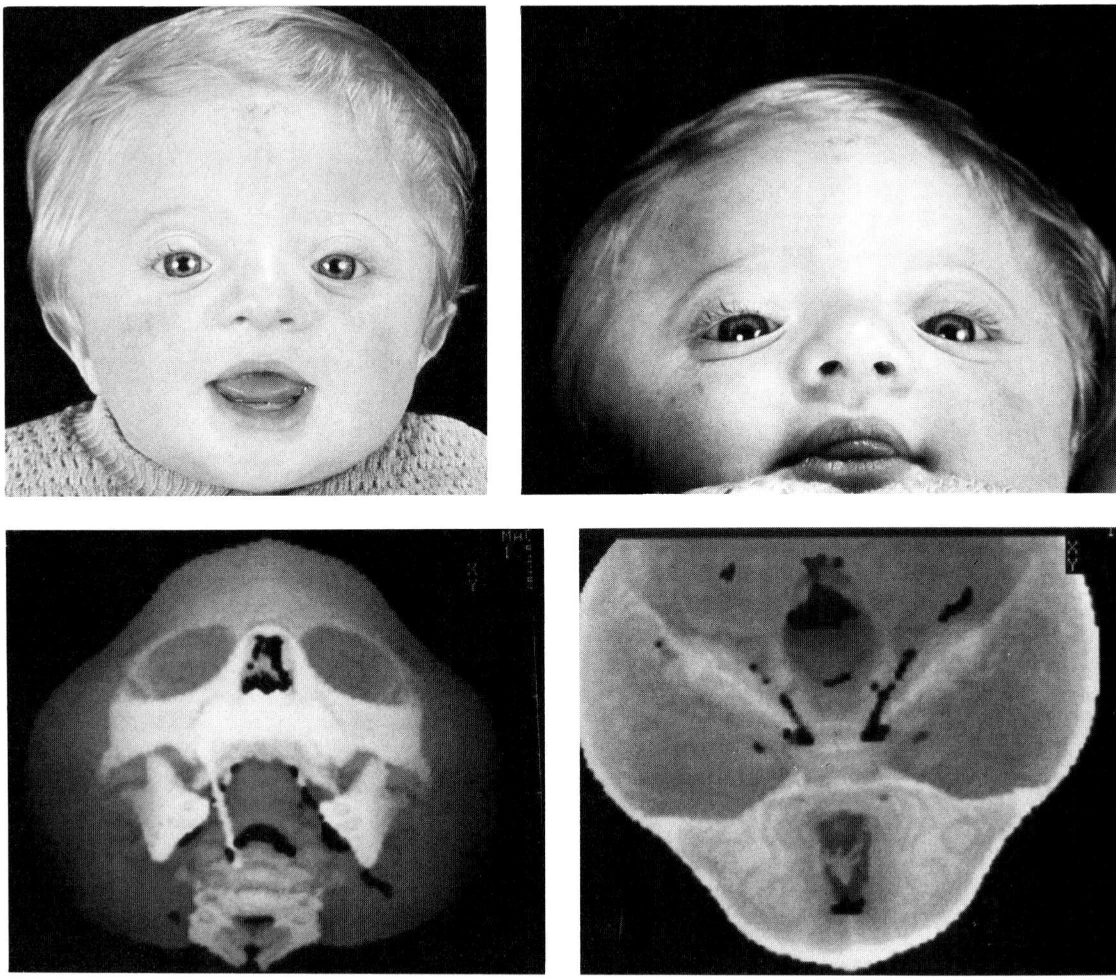

Fig. 4.3. **A** Hypotelorism and the wedge-shaped deformity of the forehead are characteristic of trigonocephaly. **B** Median ridge is more pronounced when viewed from below. **C** Central prominence slopes away to lateral forehead recessions. **D** Lateral foreshortening of the anterior cranial fossa is clearly demonstrated with a skull base view.

Fig. 4.4. **A,B** The broad, tall head shape of turricephaly secondary to familial bicoronal synostosis is shown in an adult. **C** Lateral three-dimensional image of the man in Figure 4.4A depicts the tall forehead and an obtuse frontonasal angle. **D,E** The son of the patient in Figure 4.4A displays facial features of bicoronal synostosis, similar to those of his father. **F** Fusing left coronal suture is apparent in the son's three-dimensional image. ▶

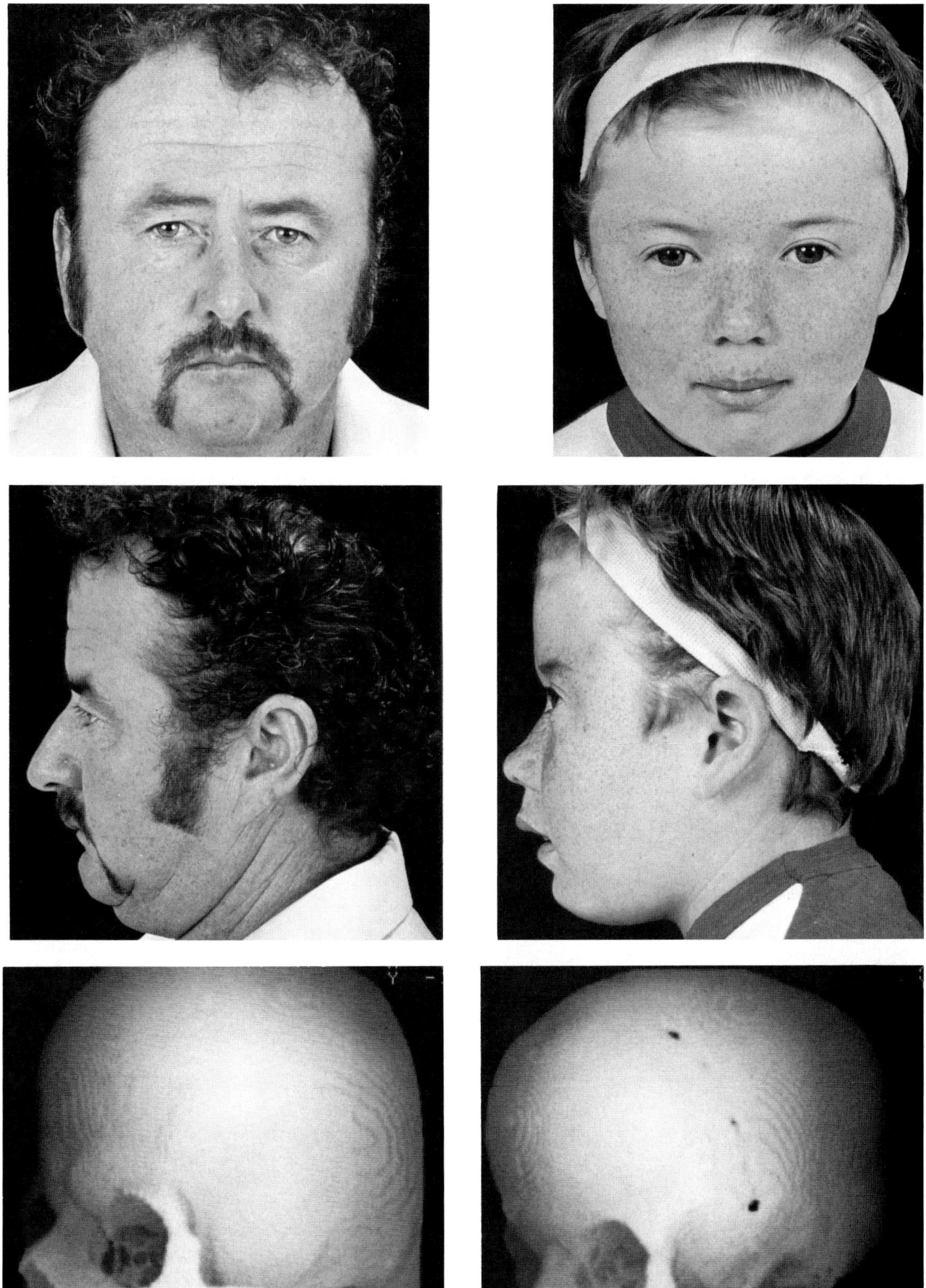

A B C D E F

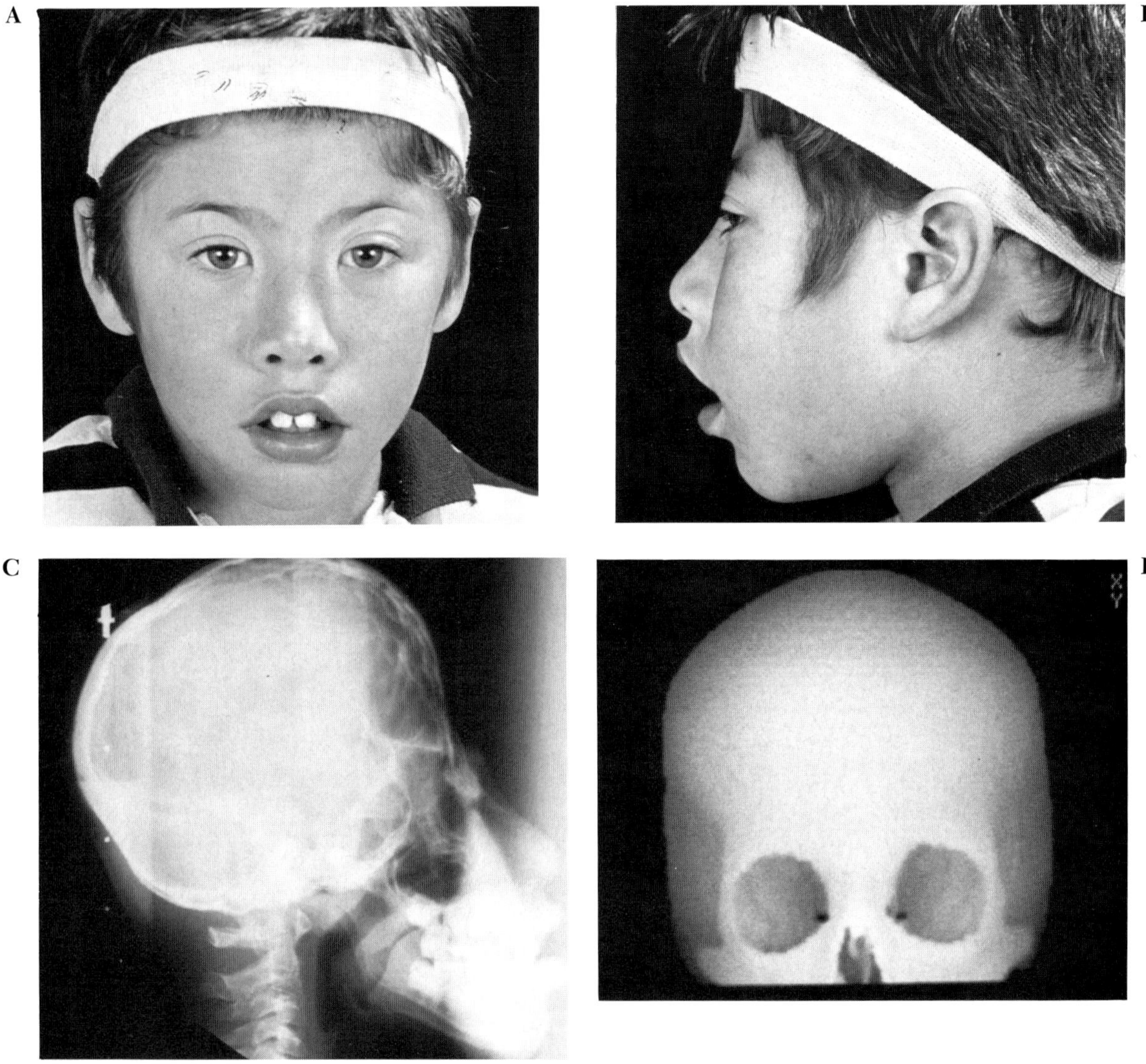

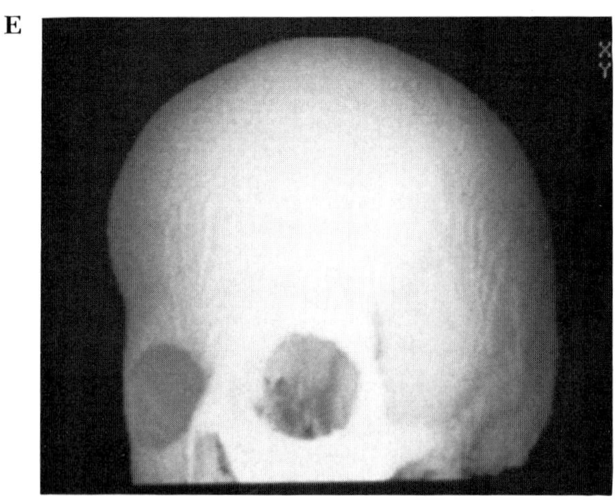

Fig. 4.5. A,B Typical appearance of turricephaly is a flattened, almost concave forehead, recessed supraorbital margins, and obtuse frontonasal angle. **C** Lateral cephalometric radiograph shows the distorted skull with some copper beating, orbitostenosis particularly affecting the upper orbit, obtuse frontonasal angle, and relatively normal lower face. **D** Skull is tower-shaped with widening of the intercanthal distance and broadening of the interorbital distance resulting in mild hypertelorism. **E** No coronal suture can be seen in the left lateral oblique view, but there is obvious flattening of the forehead and supraorbital margins.

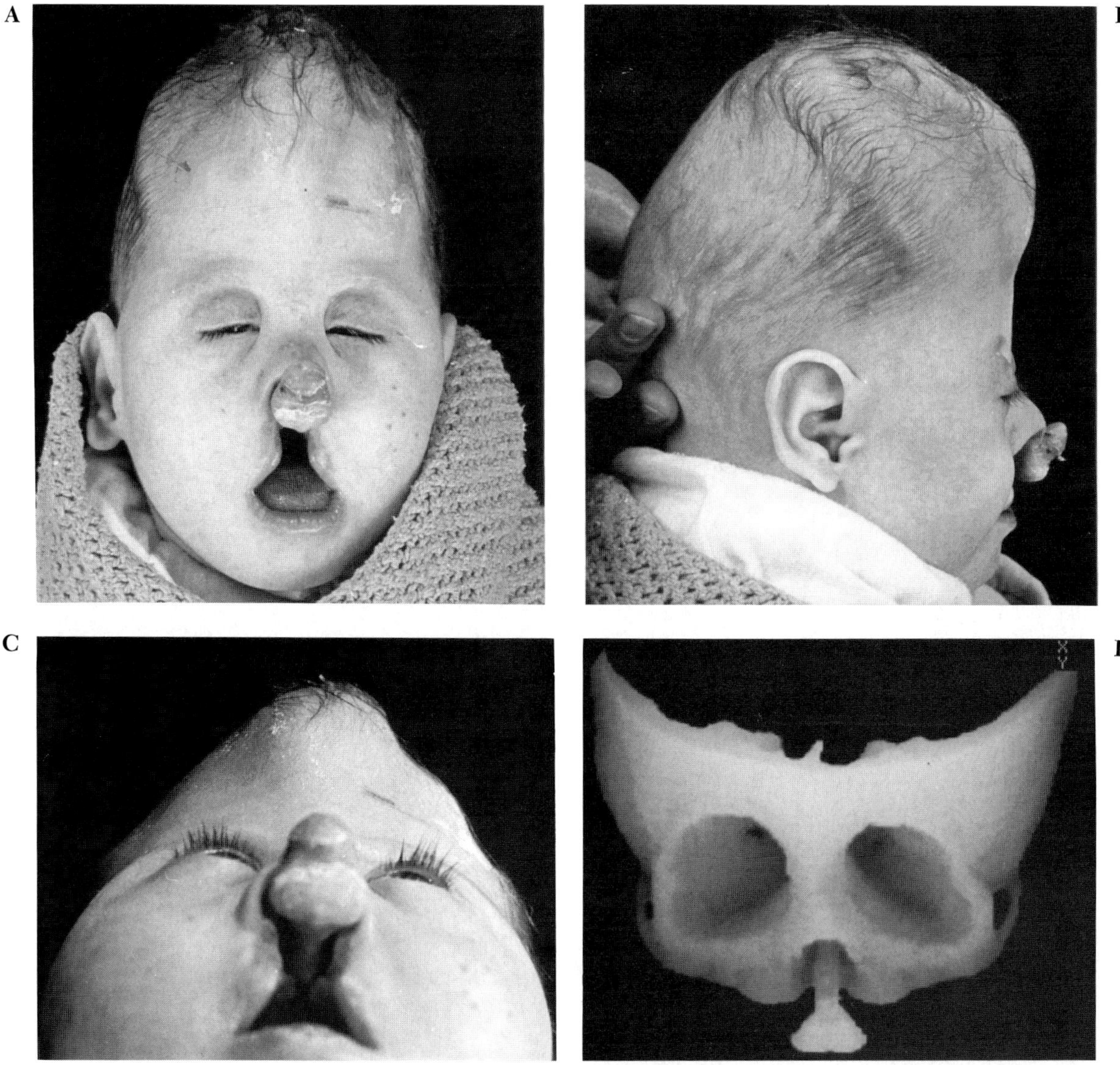

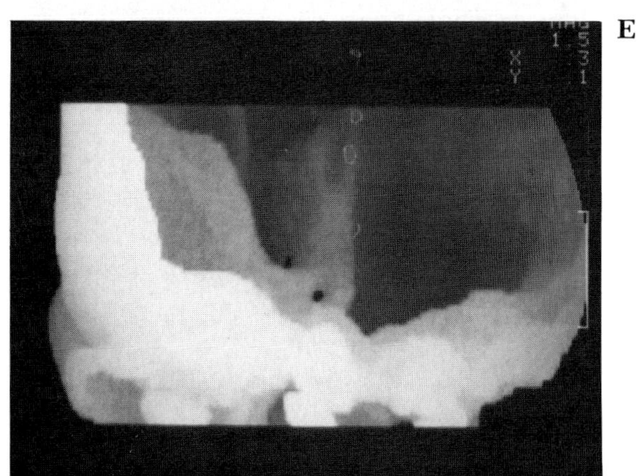

Fig. 4.6. A–C Pointed oxycephalic head shape is obvious in this patient with complex craniosynostosis. Hypotelorism and bilateral cleft lip and palate deformities are also seen. **D** Orbital elongation and the skeletal deformity of a bilateral cleft are well demonstrated. **E** From the posterior aspect, the view from the middle cranial fossa looking into the anterior cranial fossa is limited by the swept-up sphenoidal ridges around a distorted anterior cranial fossa with a depressed cribriform plate.

A

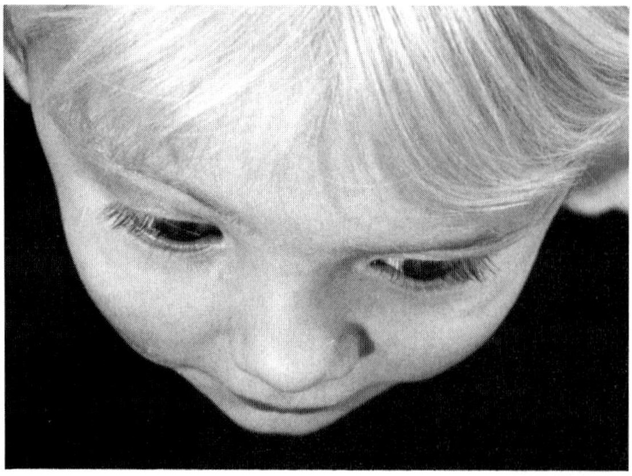

B

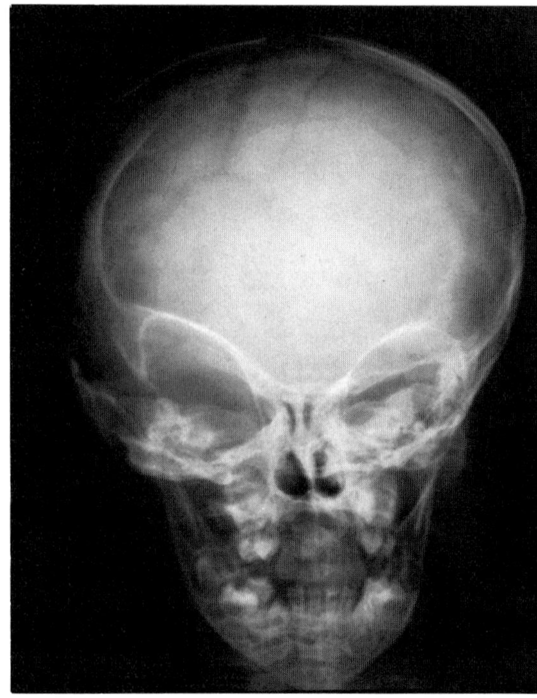

C

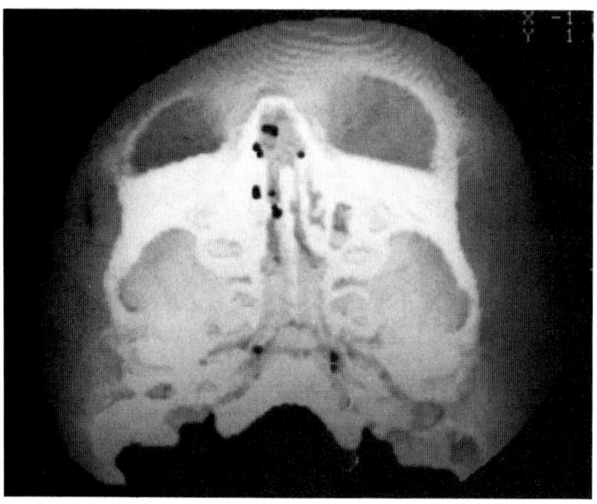

D

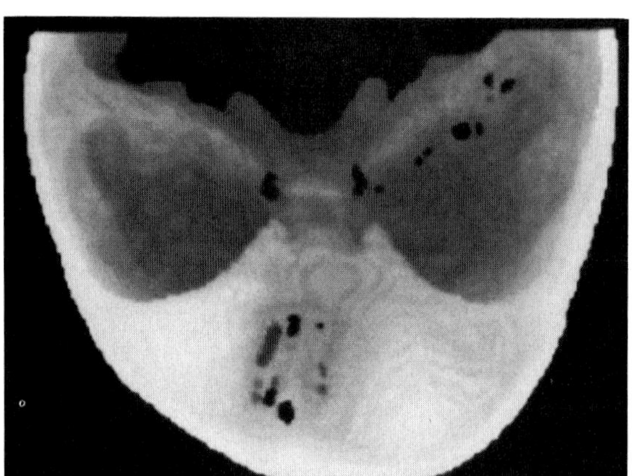

Fig. 4.7. A Frontal plagiocephaly is most obvious when the eyebrow positions are compared by viewing the patient from above. **B** Premature fusion of a coronal suture with a swept-up sphenoidal ridge produces the typical plain radiographic appearance of a harlequin orbit. **C** Frontal and orbital asymmetry are obvious with the three-dimensional image in a submental projection. **D** Widening of the cribriform plate and shortening of the anterior cranial fossa and the middle fossa on the affected side are features that are best viewed with the internal base view.

A
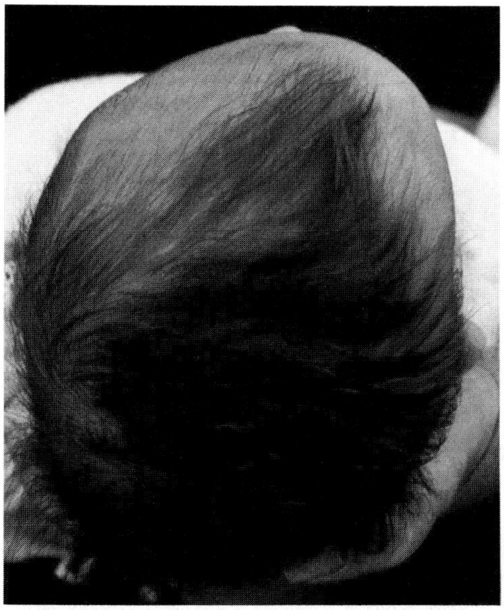

B
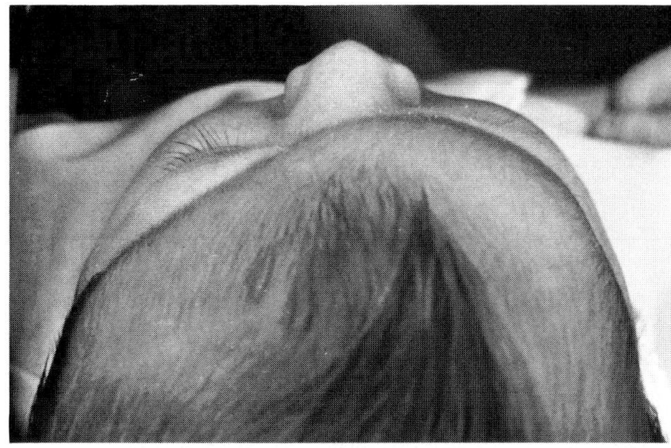

C
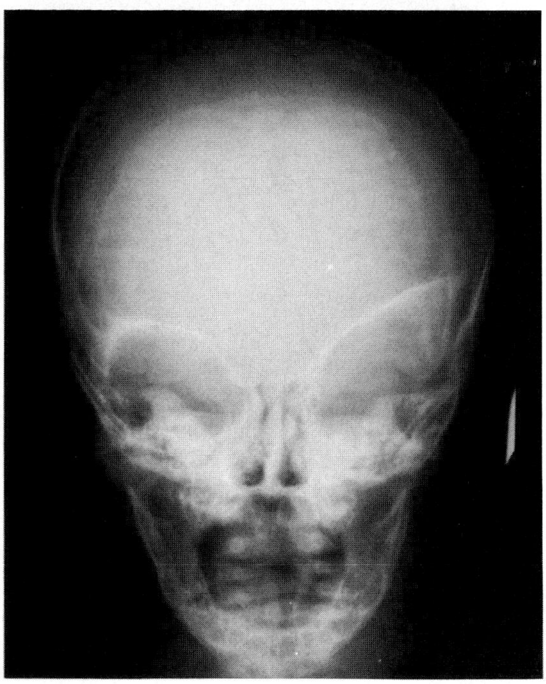

D
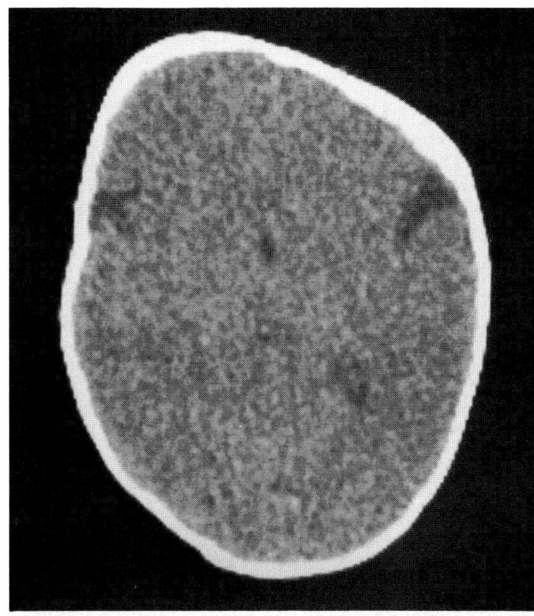

E
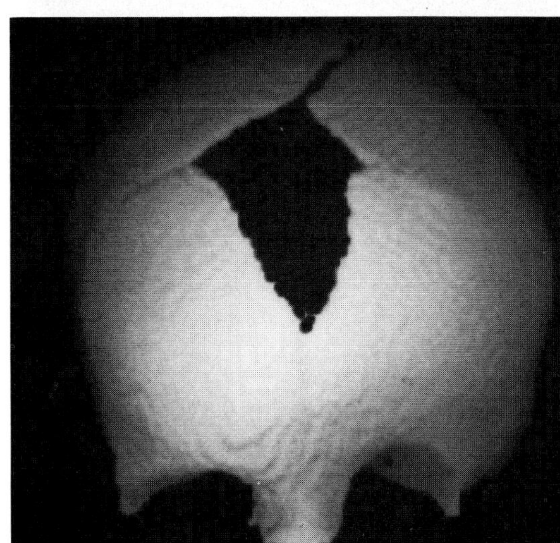

Fig. 4.8. A,B Plagiocephaly. There is flattening of the left frontal and right occipital regions. **C** Plain radiograph demonstrates the harlequin orbit on the left side. **D** Parallelogram head shape with normal underlying brain is demonstrated in the standard CT axial slice. **E** The fused coronal suture on the left and the patent suture on the right are associated with shape distortion of the anterior fontanelle. The left orbit is swept up, and there is asymmetry of the root of the nose.

A D B E C F

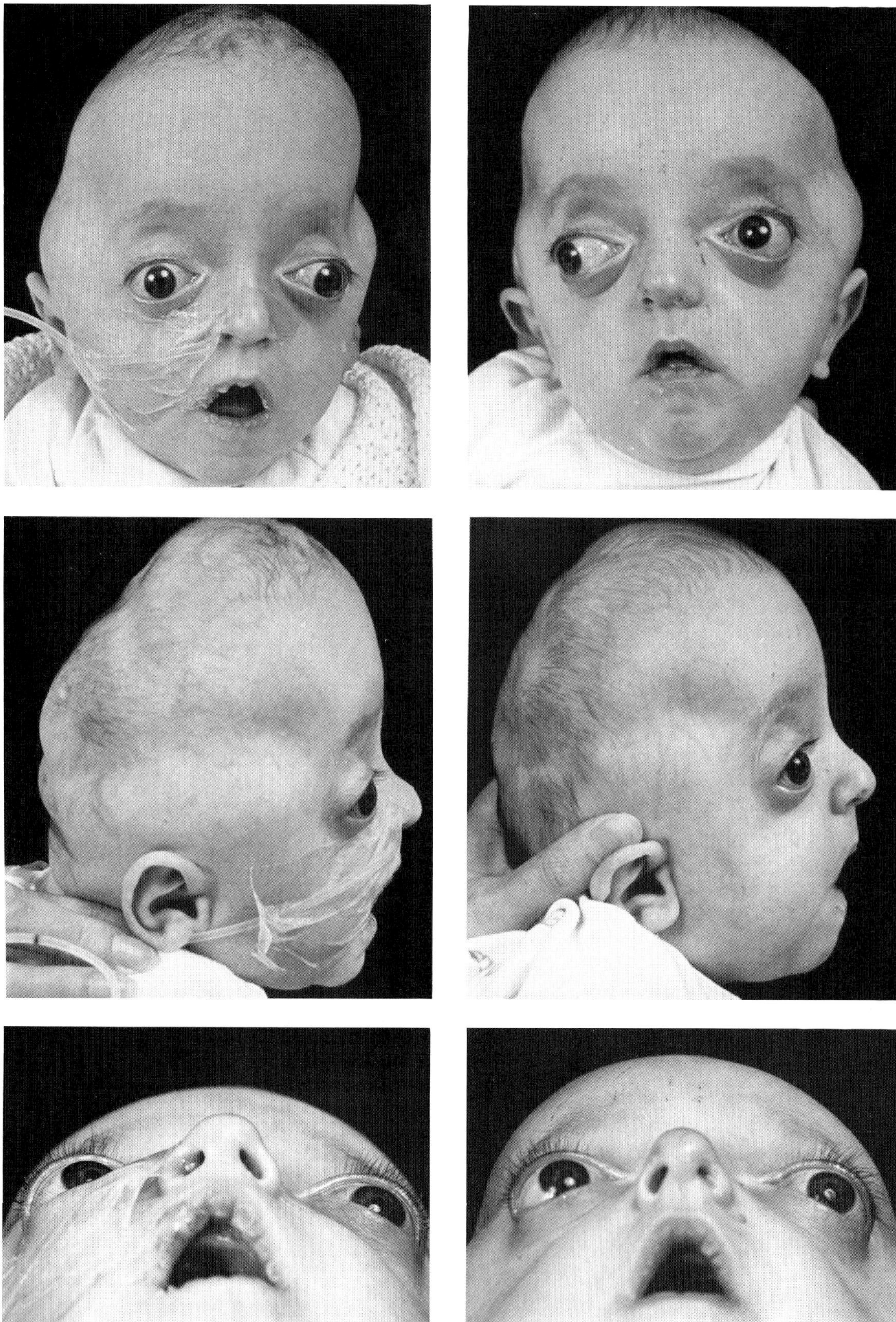

G

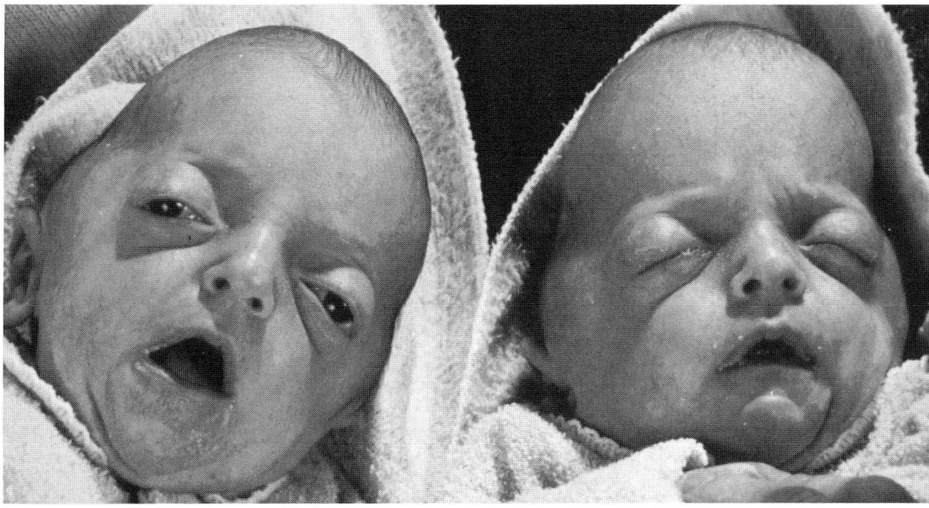

H

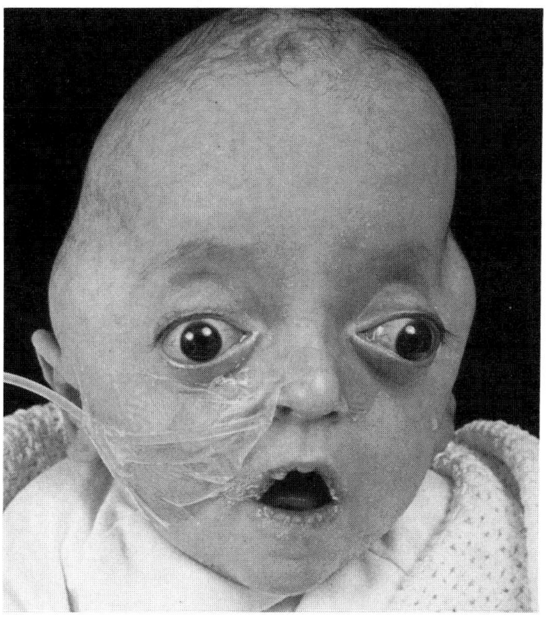

I

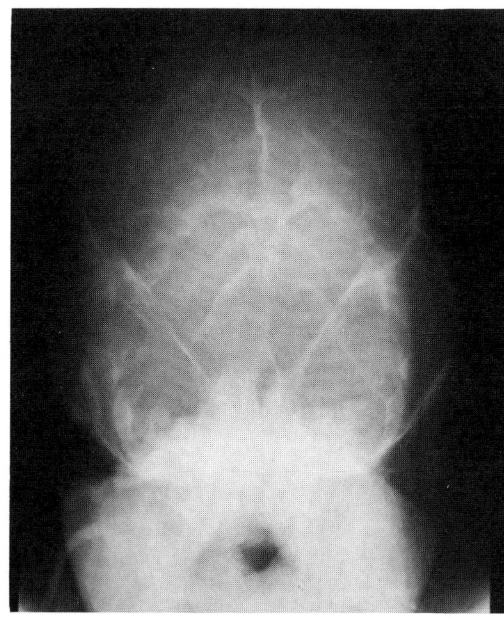

Fig. 4.9. A–C Twin 1 with Crouzon syndrome. The skull is grossly distorted and is more oxycephalic than that of twin 2. **D–F** Twin 2. Multiple sutural fusion has caused depressions in the temporal regions with a resulting triphyllocephalic head shape. Orbitostenosis has caused extrusion of the eyeballs with a marked divergent squint. **G** Twins with severe Crouzon syndrome show the typical features of triphyllocephaly with bulging of the middle cranial fossa, exorbitism, and hypoplasia of the midface. **H** Twin 1. **I** Plain skull radiograph of twin 1 demonstrates the triphyllocephalic deformity and evidence of raised intracranial pressure. **J** The swept-up distortion of the shallow orbits is apparent on the three-dimensional image, which also shows evidence of a patent sagittal suture and bone thinning in the temporal regions. **K** On lateral view the bizarre head shape is obvious. Raised intracranial pressure has caused thinning of bone. It is not well imaged owing to partial volume averaging. **L** Twin 2. **M** Plain radiograph of twin 2 shows a head shape similar to that of twin 1. **N** Marked orbitostenosis and resulting exorbitism are well demonstrated in this axial slice. **O** Three-dimensional image shows upward extrusion of the shallow orbits and the "cloverleaf" head shape. **P** Deformities similar to those of twin 1. The parietal pseudoforamina are more evident, and the degree of midface hypoplasia is severe. **J–P** See pp. 48 and 49.

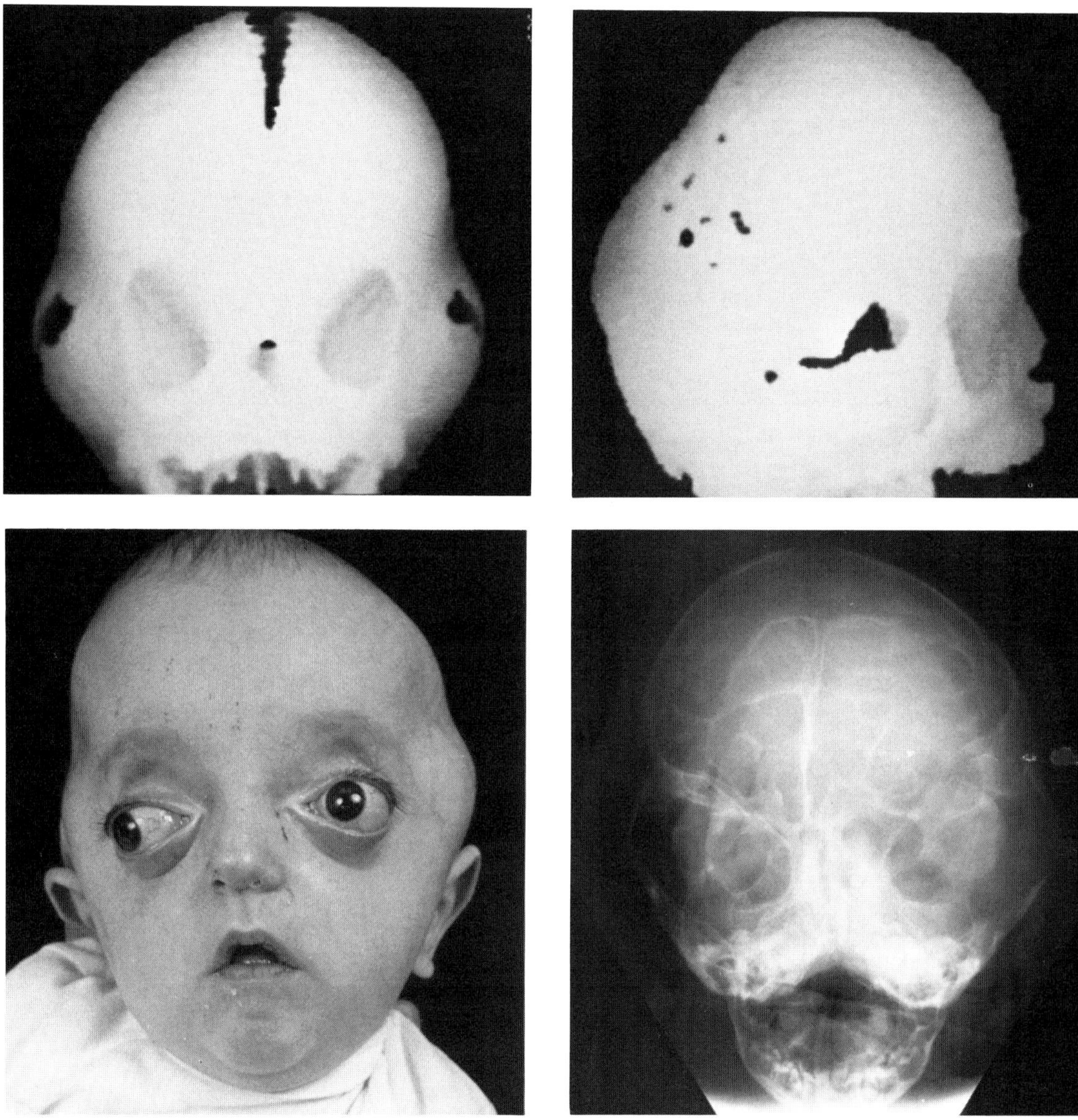

Fig. 4.9 (contd)

N

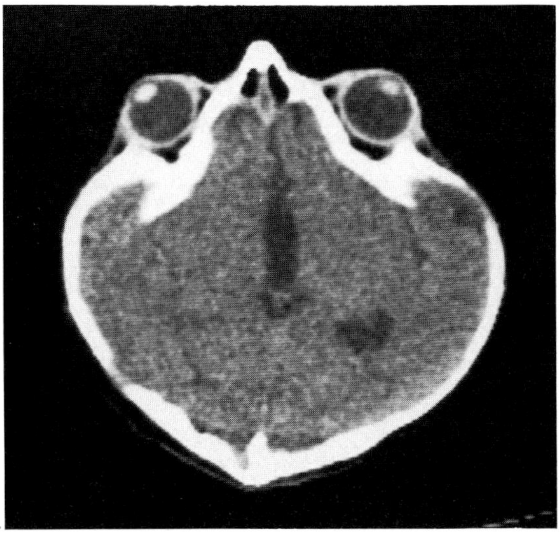

O

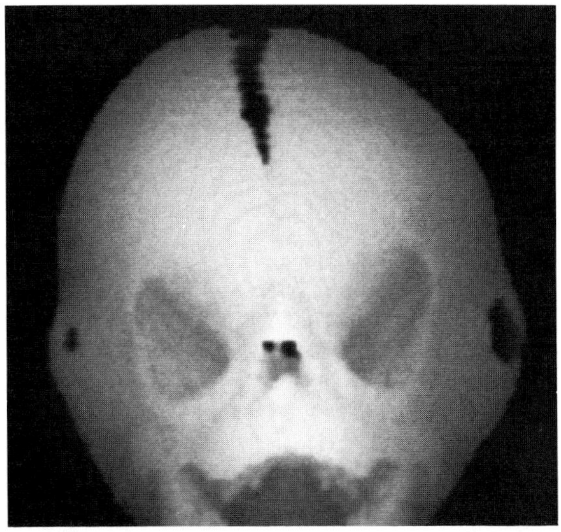

P

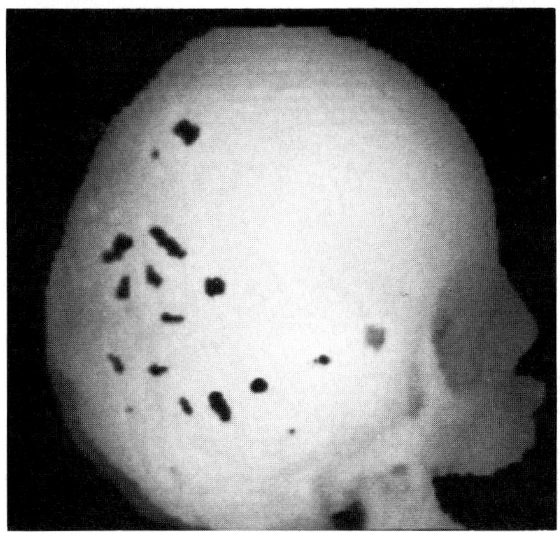

Fig. 4.9 (contd)

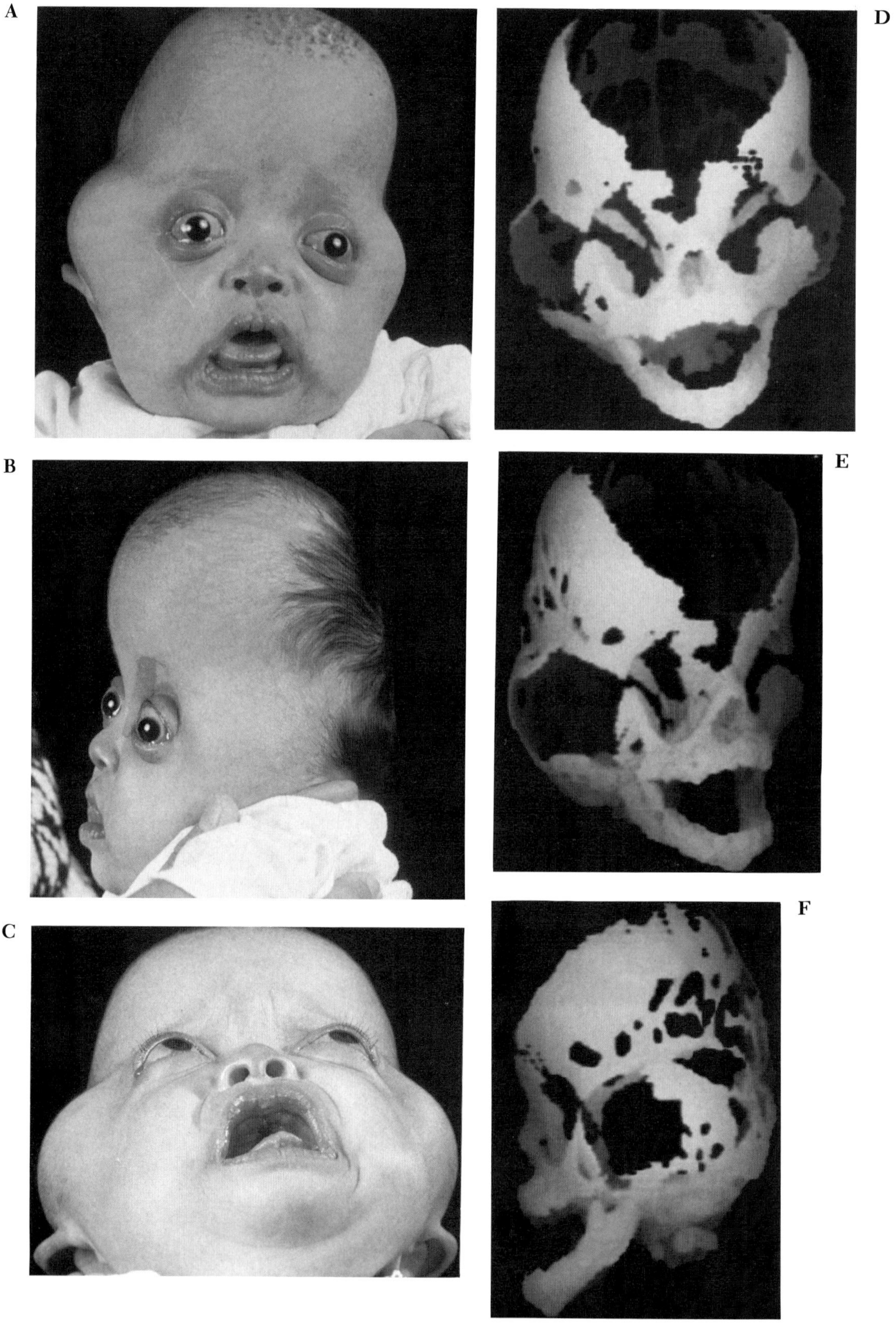
A
B
C
D
E
F

A B C D

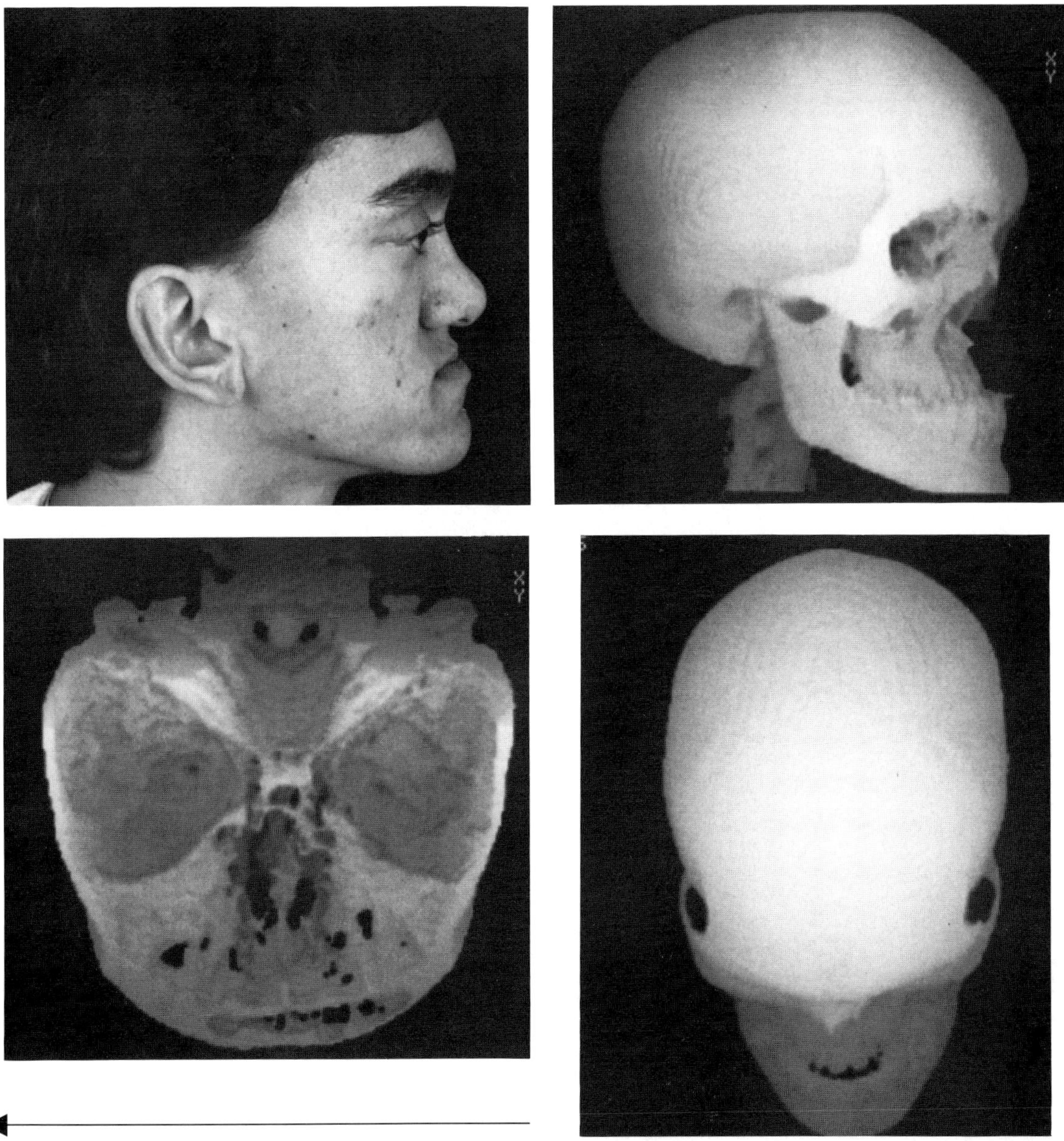

Fig. 4.10. A–C Crouzon syndrome. The cloverleaf deformity of triphyllocephaly is associated with ocular hypertelorism, proptosis, maxillary hypoplasia, and low set ears. **D** Absence of bony continuity in this three-dimensional image reflects the severity of the hydrocephalus with resultant cerebral bulging. It is not artifact. **E** Bulging outward by the temporal, and upward by the frontoparietal, regions of the brain is a consequence of the bony constriction ring between these regions. **F** Turribrachycephaly and maxillary hypoplasia are demonstrated with a lateral three-dimensional image.

Fig. 4.11. A This young adult with Crouzon syndrome has a relatively normal skull shape but severe orbitostenosis and marked midface hypoplasia with resultant class III malocclusion. **B** Recession of the inferior orbital margins contributes to the orbitostenosis. There is impressive maxillary hypoplasia and fasciostenosis. **C** This anterior cranial fossa has relatively normal dimensions. **D** The skull shape is normal, but midface recession and malocclusion are present.

A

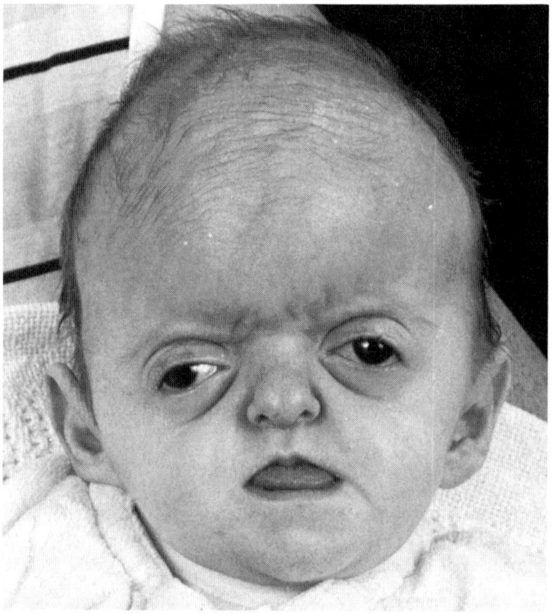

B

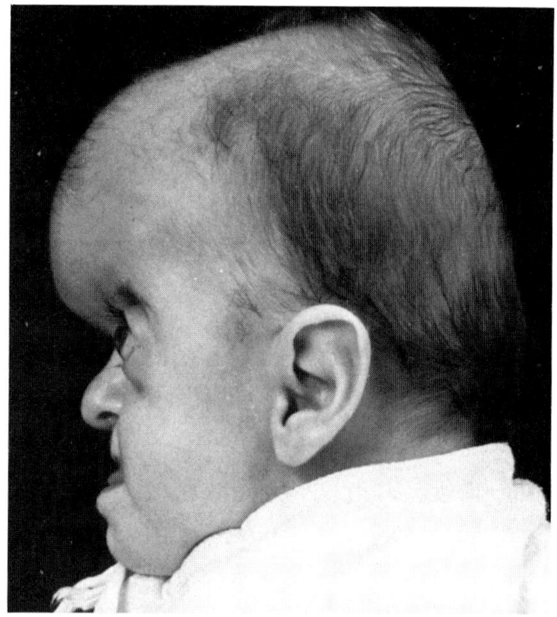

C

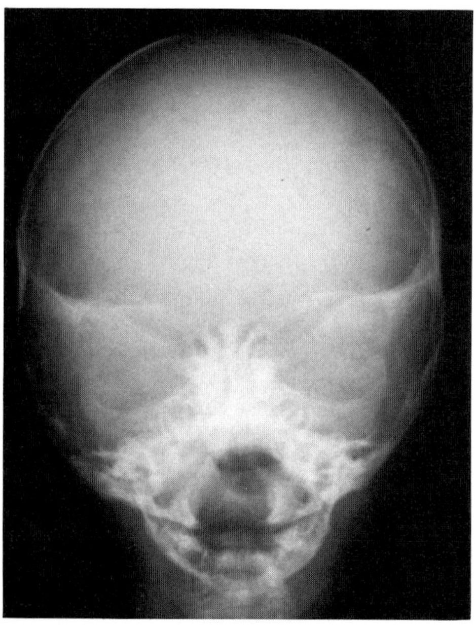

Fig. 4.12. A,B Craniofacial deformity of severe Apert syndrome in a baby. **C** Swept-up appearance of the sphenoidal ridges and a small midface. **D** Widely patent anterior fontanelle and patent sagittal suture. Bilateral ridges appear at the site of the prematurely fused coronal sutures. There is a marked disproportion between the maxilla and mandible. **E** The maxilla is markedly hypoplastic. Zygomatic bones, although small, are less severely affected.

D E

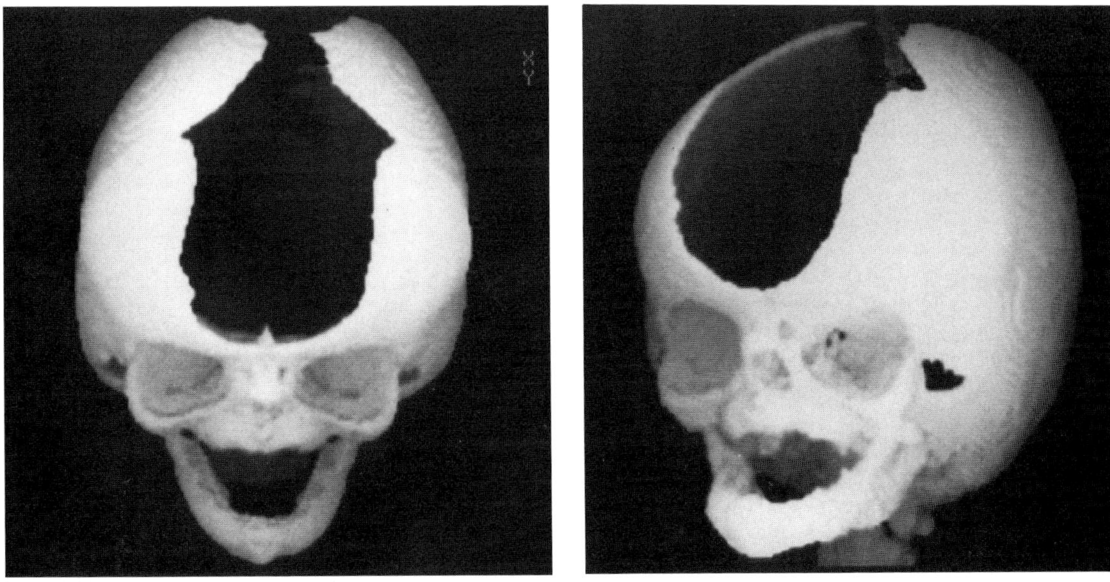

Fig. 4.12 (contd)

A B

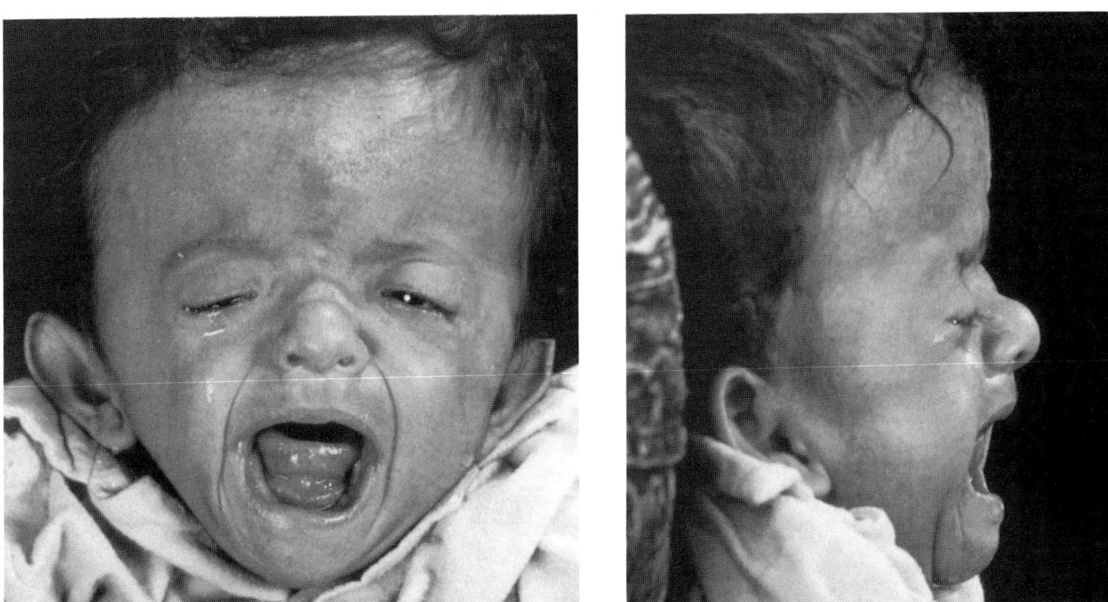

Fig. 4.13. A,B Small, retruded face of Apert syndrome. Note the recessed supraorbital ridges, small midface, and relatively prognathic mandible. **C–F** All bony features of an infant with Apert syndrome can be seen. They include turribrachycephaly, wide open fontanelle, patent metopic suture, orbital hypertelorism, maxillary hypoplasia with retrodisplaced zygomas, and relative prominence of the mandible. **C–F** See p. 54.

C D E F

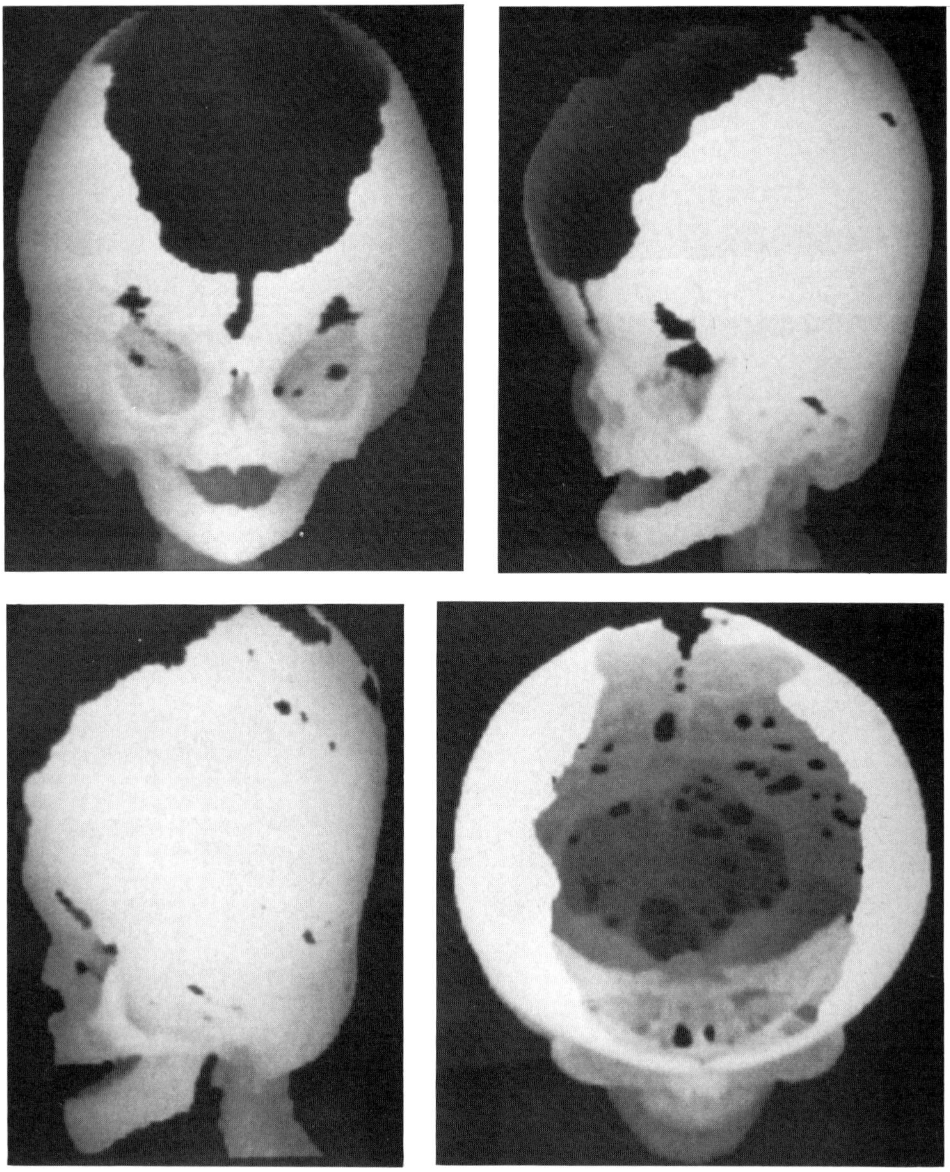

Fig. 4.13 (contd)

Fig. 4.14. A,B Child with untreated Apert syndrome who has turricephaly, exorbitism, and midface hypoplasia. **C** The most striking abnormalities on the plain skull radiograph include evidence of raised intracranial pressure, distorted orbits, and a small maxilla. **D** Severe brachycephaly can be appreciated with a lateral three-dimensional image view, which also

A

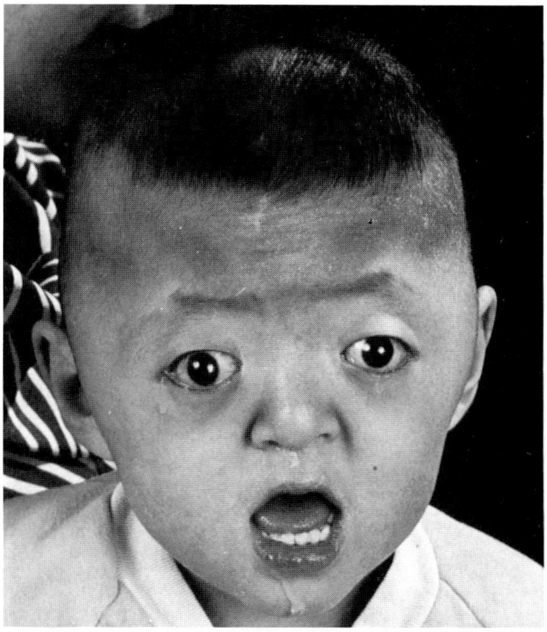

B

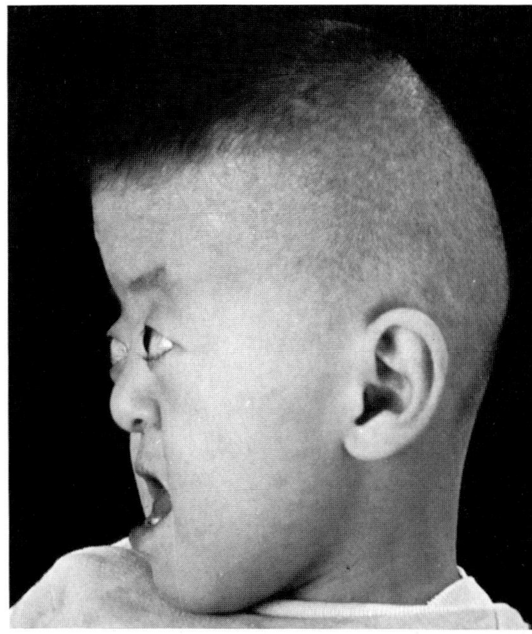

C

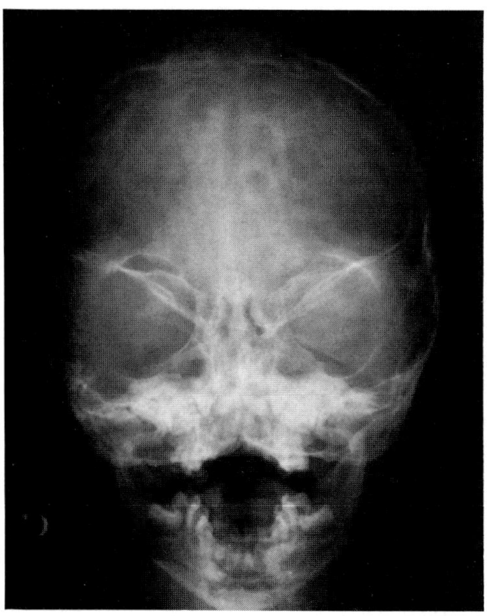

D

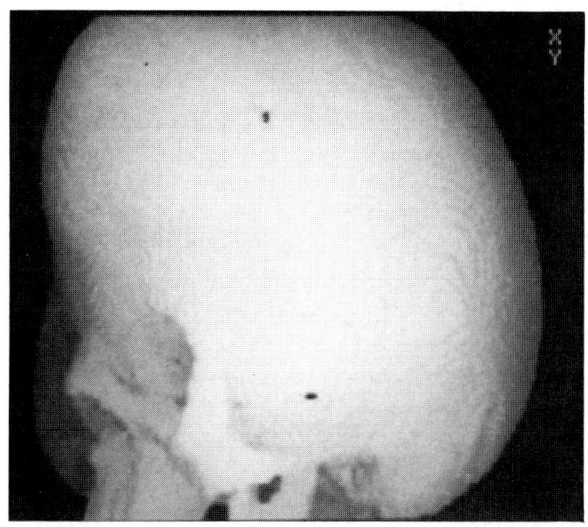

E

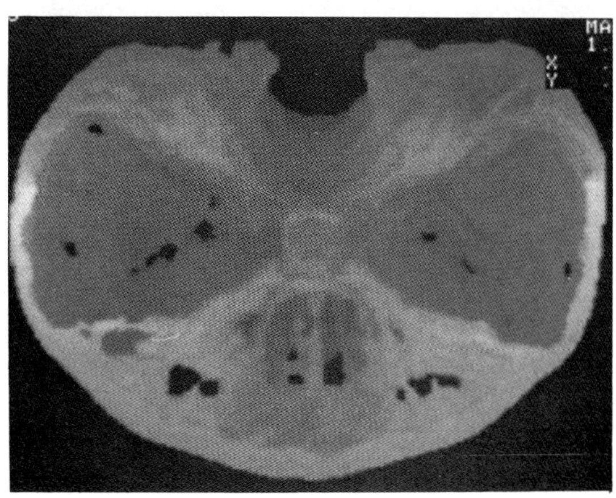

shows the anterior fontanelle to be closed at this stage. Zygomatic bones tilt downward to articulate with the hypoplastic maxilla. **E** Foreshortened anterior cranial fossa contains a depressed cribriform plate that is broadened and has a prominent crista galli. Stalagmites projecting up into the dura are typical of craniosynostosis. There is a forward projection of the middle cranial fossa laterally.

A B

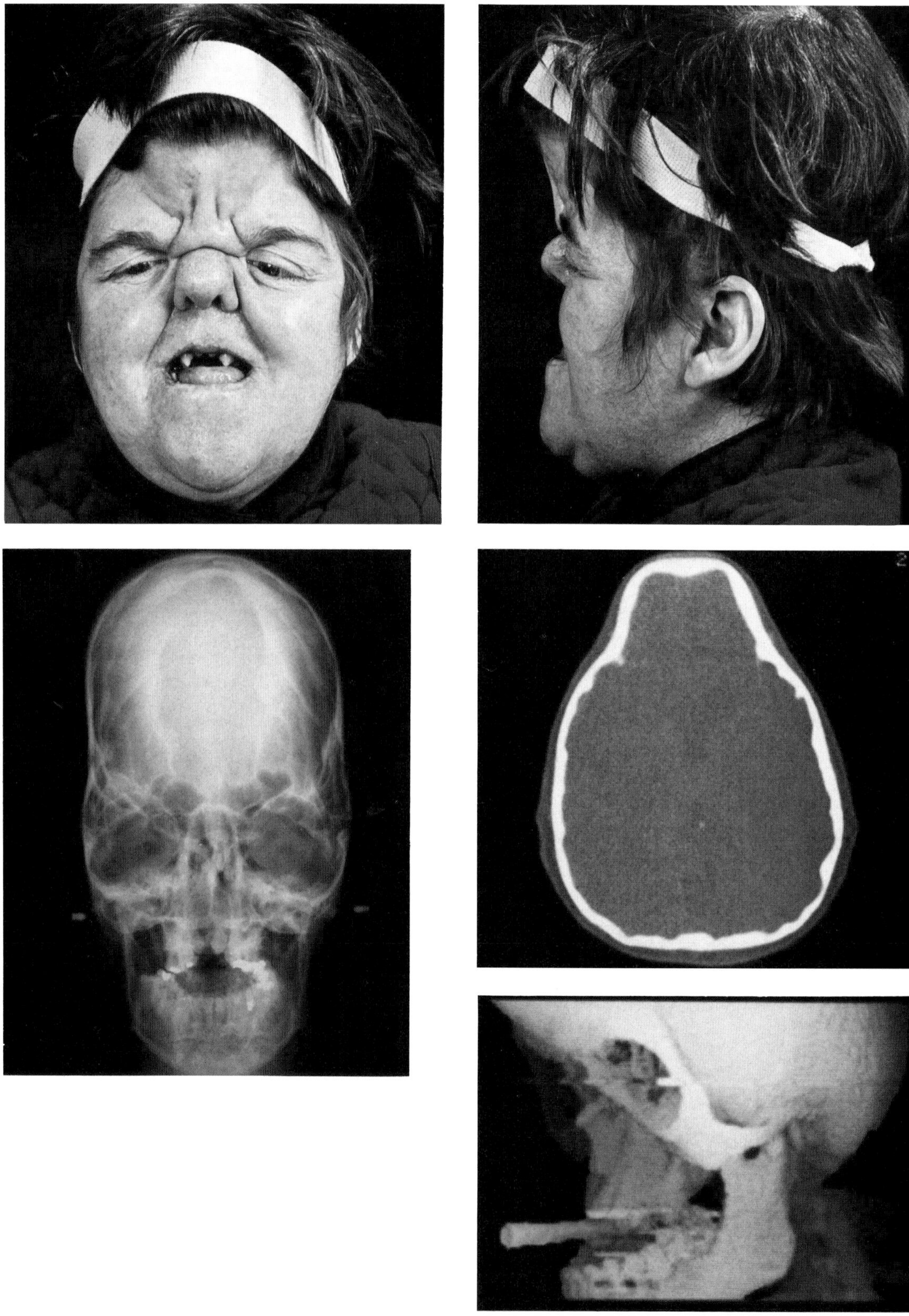

C D E

F

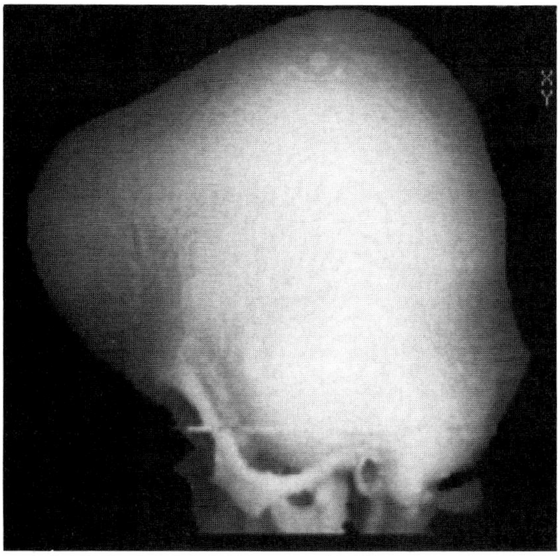

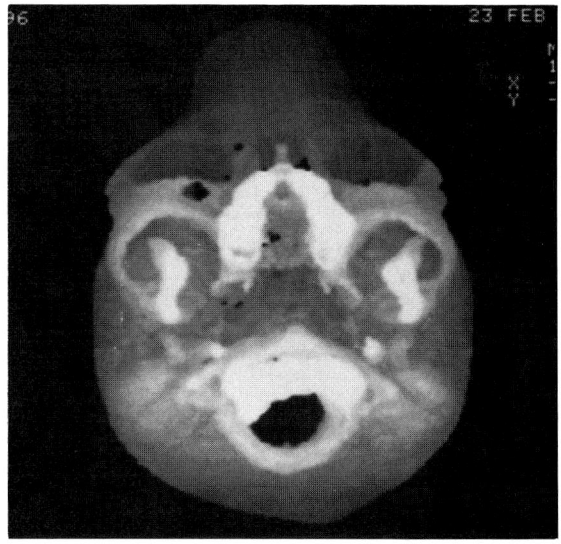

G

Fig. 4.15. A,B Adult with untreated Apert syndrome. **C** Note the turricephaly, orbital distortion, and midface hypoplasia with a resulting anterior open bite. **D** Contracted anterior cranial fossa and underlying brain of normal appearance. **E** The tiny maxilla is striking, and there are virtually no nasal bones. Note the typical distortion of the zygomatic bone, which is relatively normal in its posterior and lateral aspects but appears to be restricted in its forward growth. It results in a distorted orbit that slopes downward and backward. (Endotracheal tube is projecting from the mouth.) **F** Gross distortion of the skull is obvious with a lateral view. Note the marked bregmatic prominence in this patient. **G** Viewed from below, the distorted skull and orbits are seen above the tiny maxilla, with the pterygoid plates posteriorly.

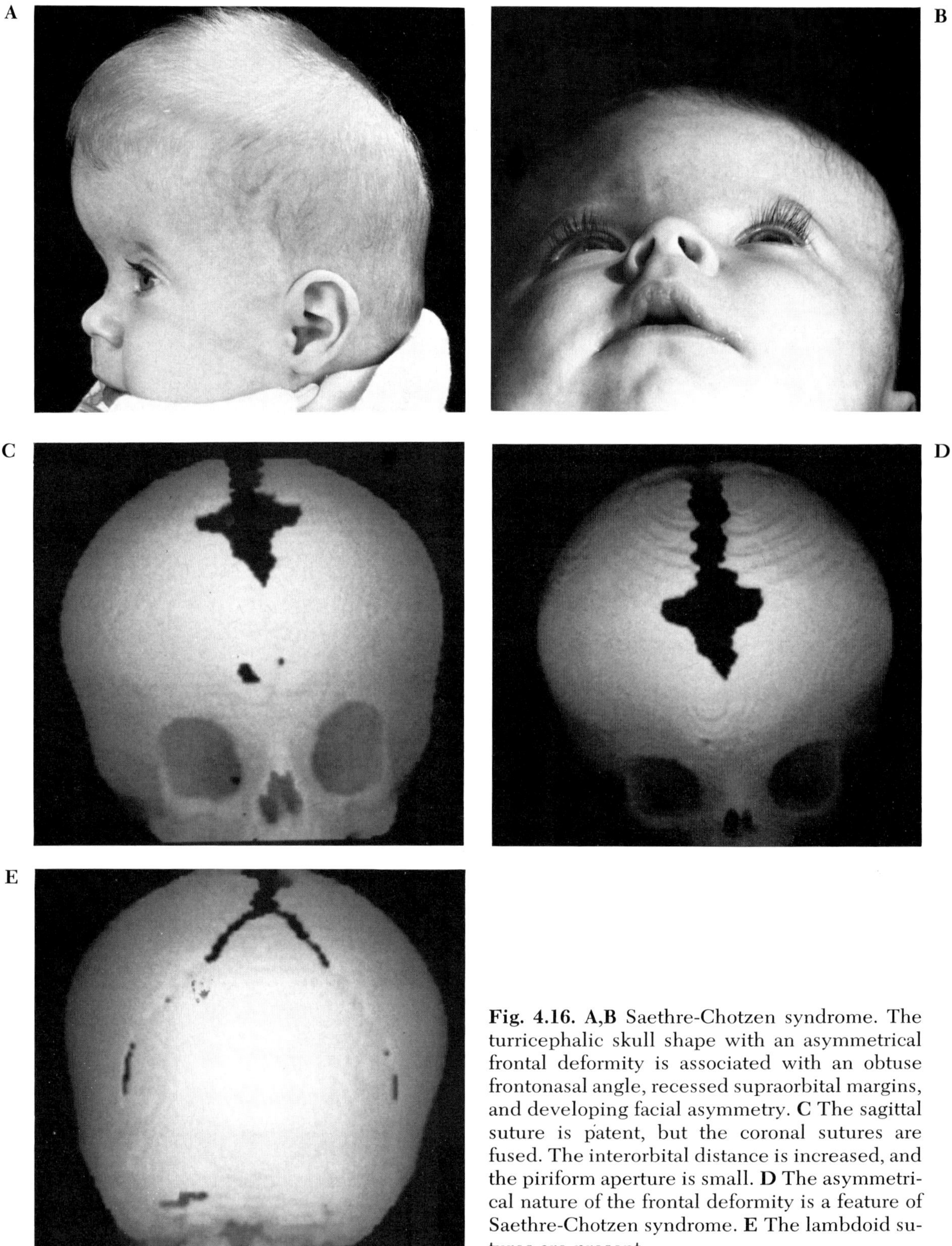

Fig. 4.16. A,B Saethre-Chotzen syndrome. The turricephalic skull shape with an asymmetrical frontal deformity is associated with an obtuse frontonasal angle, recessed supraorbital margins, and developing facial asymmetry. **C** The sagittal suture is patent, but the coronal sutures are fused. The interorbital distance is increased, and the piriform aperture is small. **D** The asymmetrical nature of the frontal deformity is a feature of Saethre-Chotzen syndrome. **E** The lambdoid sutures are present.

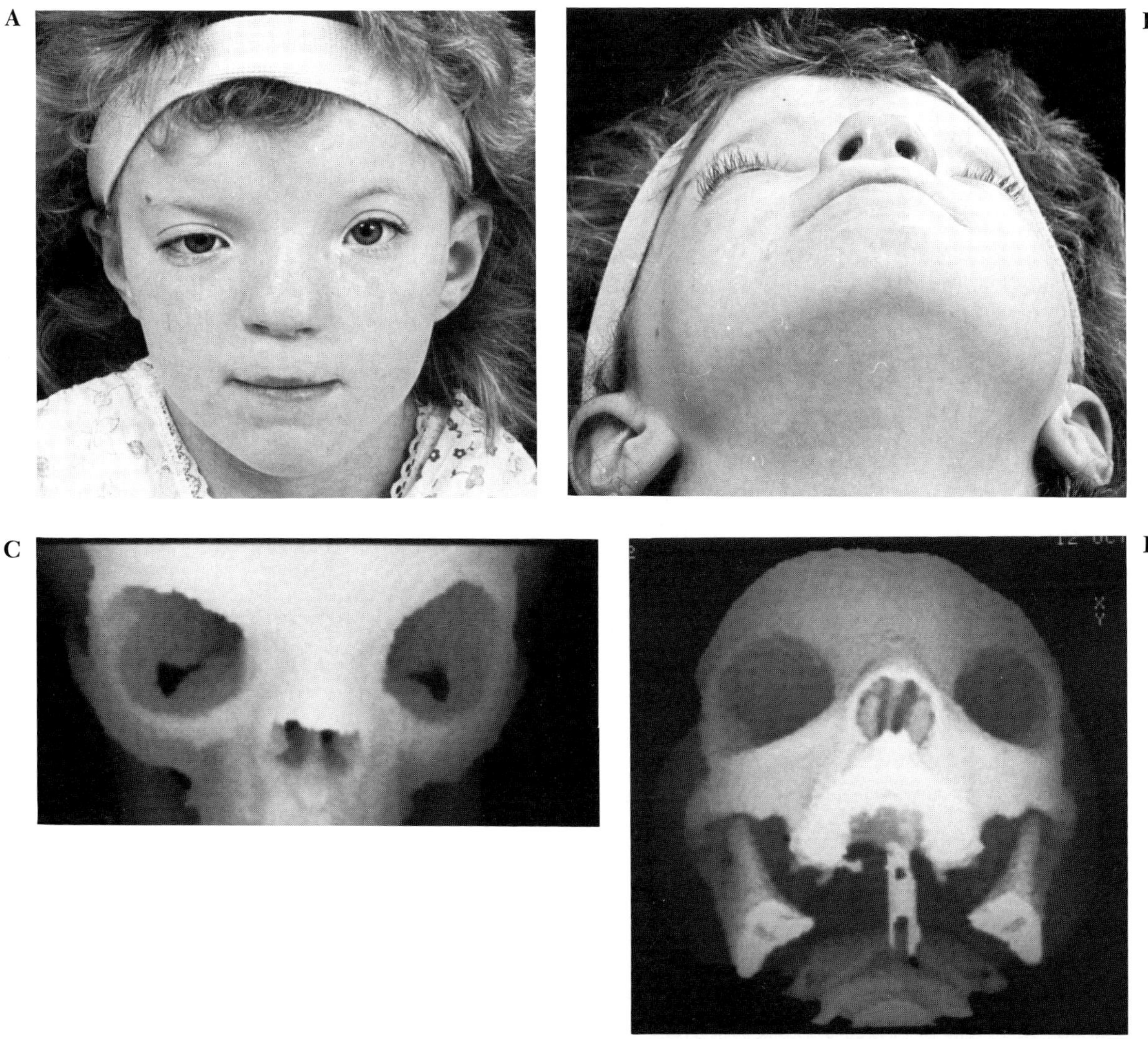

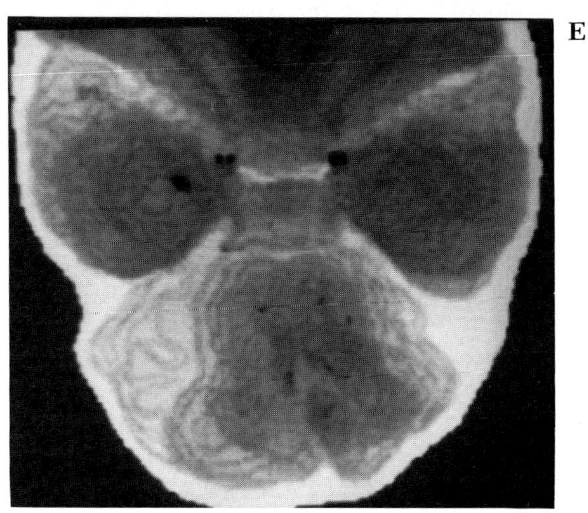

Fig. 4.17. A,B The obvious clinical features of Cohen syndrome include hypertelorism and a bifid nose. **C** The degree of hypertelorism is well demonstrated with a three-dimensional image. **D** Flattening of the left frontoorbital region, a microform of the bifid nose, and the increased interorbital distance can be further appreciated in the submental projection. **E** The anterior cranial fossa is distorted, and the cribriform plate is depressed.

A

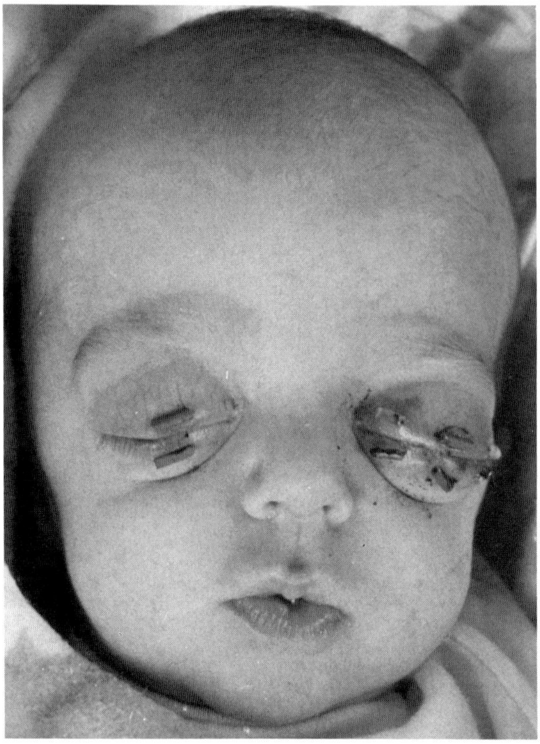

B

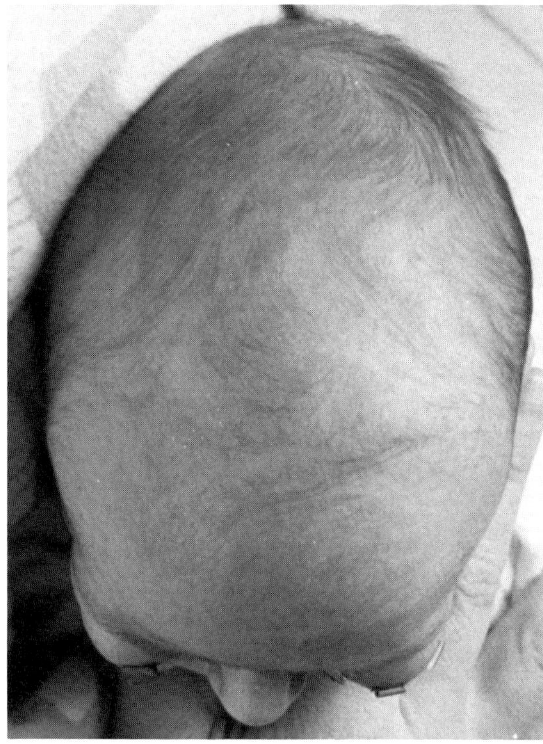

C

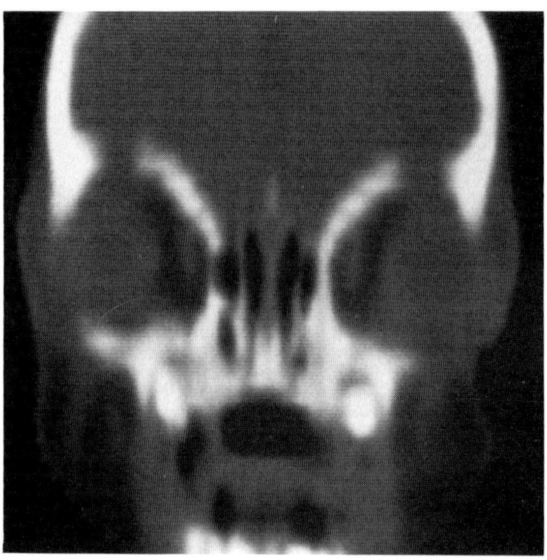

Fig. 4.18. A Pfeiffer syndrome is associated with ocular proptosis and hypertelorism. Temporary tarsorrhaphies serve to maintain the ocular globes within their shallow orbits. Note the turricephaly. **B** Viewed from above, the ocular proptosis is striking. There are ridges at the sites of the prematurely fused coronal sutures. **C** Coronal reformat illustrates well the hypoplastic maxilla. **D** The metopic suture is patent in this Pfeiffer syndrome patient. Note the widely spaced orbits and the tiny maxilla. The lower limits of the small pterygoid plates can be seen in the depths of the oral cavity. **E** The anterior fontanelle is widely open, and the metopic suture has not fused. There is no sign of the coronal sutures, which have prematurely fused and have left bony ridges.

D E

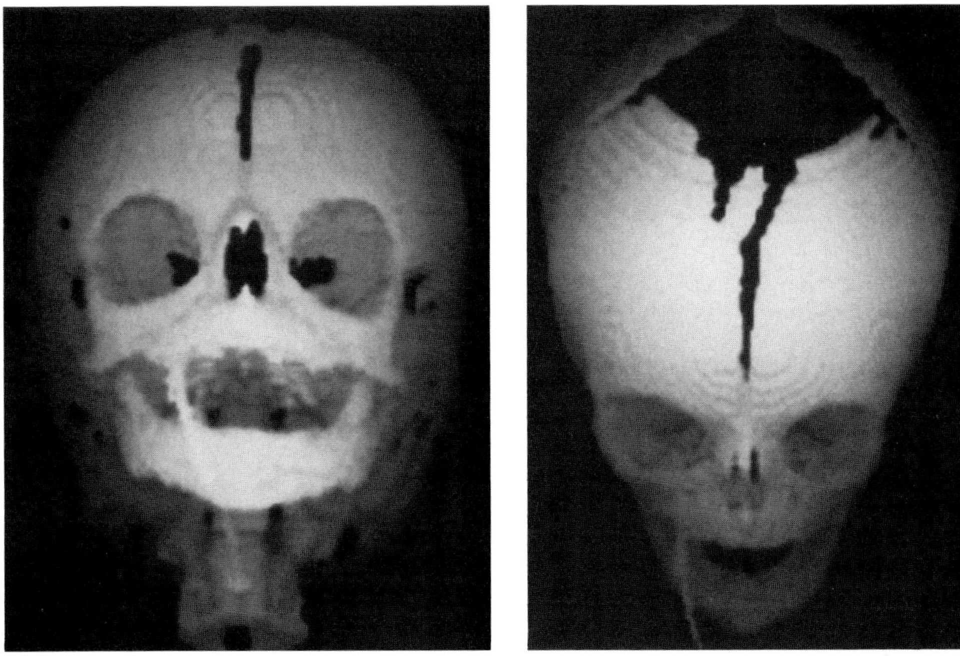

Fig. 4.18 (contd)

5

Craniofacial Clefts

Many investigators have attempted to classify craniofacial clefts, including Morian (1887), Sanvenero-Rosselli (1953), Boo-Chai (1970), Karfik (1966), Pfeifer (1974), Mazzola (1976), and van der Meulen (1985). Tessier (1976) introduced a new classification in an effort to eliminate confusing terminology and to provide a better understanding of these rare malformations.

"Tessier" Craniofacial Clefts

Tessier's classification, based on personal observation, was designed to facilitate accurate recording of these defects. A system of numbering was devised using 0 as the median facial dysraphia. Each cleft was then assigned a number determined by an axis in relation to the 0 line (Figs. 5.1–5.15). This method provides an immediate reference to the exact anatomical location, with the original numerical allocation being made after clinical examination and surgical dissections. Three-dimensional imaging offers an opportunity to study the proposition that craniofacial clefts are reflected in distortions of cranial base anatomy, especially in the sphenoid bone. Such imaging provides both scientist and clinician with a technique for developing greater insight into cleft pathology. Although a cleft may be tracked with two-dimensional reformats, three-dimensional imaging presents an overall picture of the shape distortion, especially with views of the cranial base distortion.

Cleft 0 is a cleft through the frontal bone, crista galli, and midline of the nose. It may extend through the columella, lip, and maxilla (Figs. 5.13–5.15).

Cleft 1 goes through the frontal bone, along the nasoorbital nerve, through the olfactory groove of the cribriform plate, and then between the nasal bone and frontal process of the maxilla. It extends through the dome of the alar cartilage and may involve the lip and alveolus in the form of a cleft lip (Figs. 5.1 and 5.2).

Cleft 2 is a paranasal cleft located between the tail of the alar cartilage and the alar base, extending through the lateral masses of the medial canthus (Figs. 5.1–5.3).

Cleft 3 runs from the upper lip to the lacrimal portion of the lower eyelid (Fig. 5.4). It involves clefting of the lip and alveolus, extending around the base of the ala in the nasolabial groove to the lower eyelid through the lacrimal gutter and frontal process of the maxilla.

Cleft 4 passes between the upper lip and the lower eyelid, remaining medial to the infraorbital nerve (Fig. 5.5). It passes through the lip midway between the philtral crest and the labial commissure. However, the cleft in the alveolus always corresponds in position with that of a cleft palate.

Cleft 5 extends from a region of the upper lip just medial to the corner of the mouth and passes up to the lower eyelid, remaining lateral to the infraorbital nerve (Fig. 5.6). It passes through the alveolus in the premolar region.

Clefts 6, 7, and 8 are found in combination in Treacher Collins syndrome (Figs. 5.9, and 5.16–5.18). *Cleft 6* includes a coloboma of the lower eyelid between the middle and lateral third (Fig. 5.7) and a cleft between the maxilla and zygomatic bone with a soft tissue furrow that may extend to the corner of the mouth in the direction of the angle of the mandible. With *cleft 7* the zygomatic arch is usually absent, and the condyle, coronoid process, and mandibular ramus have varying degrees of deformity. Also associated with this cleft are ear malformations and a tongue of hair extending onto the cheek in Treacher Collins syndrome. Hemifacial microsomia is represented by No. 7 type clefting (Figs. 5.8 and 5.19–5.24). *Cleft 8* is characterized by absence of the lateral orbital wall and there is lateral canthal dystopia.

Cleft 9 involves the lateral one-third of the upper eyelid and supraorbital ridge.

Cleft 10 is a median cleft of the supraorbital ridge, frontal bone, and orbital roof passing lateral to the supraorbital nerve. It may be associated with colobomata of the eyebrow or upper eyelid (Fig. 5.10).

Cleft 11, in addition to extending through the frontal bone, frontal sinus, and lateral mass of the ethmoid, is associated with a coloboma of the inner one-third of the upper eyelid.

Cleft 12 is a cleft between the nasal bone and frontal process of the maxilla (Fig. 5.11). It extends through the frontal bone and the olfactory groove of the cribriform plate.

Cleft 13 is an extension into the cranial region of cleft 1 as median craniofacial dysraphia (Fig. 5.12).

Cleft 14 has been considered the cranial component of cleft 0 (Figs. 5.13–5.15).

Treacher Collins Syndrome

Treacher Collins syndrome is also known as mandibulofacial dysostosis, Berry syndrome, and Franceschetti-Zwahlen-Klein syndrome. It is transmitted by autosomal dominant inheritance with a high, but variable, penetrance and expressivity producing different degrees of involvement of affected members of the same family (Fig. 5.18E).

The patient with Treacher Collins syndrome exhibits abnormalities of the facial bones and soft tissues (Figs. 5.9 and 5.16–5.18). The fully developed syndrome consists of an antimongoloid slant of the palpebral fissures (Figs. 5.9A, 5.17A, and 5.18A), which is reflected in the underlying slope of the bony orbit (Figs. 5.9D, 5.16C, and 5.17B), and notching or colobomata of the lateral portion of the lower lids in most cases (Fig. 5.18A). Absence of the eyelashes on the medial one-third of the lower lids is a common feature (Fig. 5.18A). The bony configuration is produced in part by hypoplasia of the facial bones, always bilateral but frequently asymmetrical (Fig. 5.17B). In the complete form there is total absence of the zygomatic bones and zygomatic arches, the latter being responsible for the lack of the lateral orbital rim (Fig. 5.16C). The lateral orbital wall is formed by the hypoplastic greater wing of the sphenoid, and the inferior orbital fissure has no anterior boundary. Thus there is no separation between the orbital cavity, temporal fossa, and infratemporal fossa. The inferior orbital rim is poorly defined, and the infraorbital foramen is frequently absent, the neurovascular bundle passing directly from the orbital cavity to the cheek. The overall shape of the orbit is characteristic. There is overhanging of the lateral part of the supraorbital ridge and downward sloping of the orbital floor (Figs. 5.9C and 5.16C). The orbital contents appear to prolapse into the inferior orbital fissure.

The zygomatic arches are absent or much reduced. As a result, the aponeurosis of the hypoplastic temporalis muscle is directly continuous with the aponeurosis of the masseter muscle. According to the Tessier classification of craniofacial clefts, Treacher Collins syndrome corresponds to cleft numbers 6, 7, and 8 (Fig. 5.9).

There is typically hypoplasia of the mandible with an obtuse mandibular angle (Fig. 5.18C,D). The ramus may be deficient, and the condylar and coronoid processes may be flat or aplastic (Fig. 5.16D,E). Lower border notching is considered by some to be a specific feature of the condition (Figs. 5.16D,E and 5.18C,D).

The external ears are frequently abnormal in shape, size, and position (Figs. 5.9A, 5.16A, and 5.17A). There are often abnormalities of the middle and inner ears. There may be rudimentary ear tags, blind fistulae, or dimples between the ears and the angles of the mouth. A tongue-like projection of hair may extend onto the cheek (Fig. 5.18B).

Macrostomia (Fig. 5.16A), a high-arched palate, a receding chin (Fig. 5.18B), and an anterior open bite produce the characteristic appearance of those affected by Treacher Collins syndrome. Other associated anomalies include cleft palate (Fig. 5.16B) and deformities of the radius, ulna, metacarpals, and spine.

Craniofacial Microsomia

Craniofacial microsomia describes variable underdevelopment of the craniofacial skeleton, external ear, and facial soft tissues (Figs. 5.8, 5.19–5.24). The deformity involves structures derived from the first and second branchial arches. The term hemifacial microsomia implies unilateral facial involvement only. However, anomalies in other organ systems may occur, and both sides of the face may be involved. Facial asymmetry, phenotypic characteristics, and the lack of inheritance patterns differentiate the bilateral form of craniofacial microsomia from Treacher Collins syndrome.

The wide range of phenotypes has resulted in difficulties with classification and arguments over etiology. Mandibular deformities may range from a reduction in height (Figs. 5.19C–F) to severe malformation with complete agenesis of the ramus (Figs. 5.23H and 5.24D). If extensive, there may be orbital hypoplasia or even an asymmetrical neurocranium (Fig. 5.24). The auricle may be normal, but more often there is microtia of varying degrees, with anotia in some cases. Soft tissue defects are also variable, with major deformities resulting in facial scoliosis and severe hypoplasia of the cranial nerves, the parotid gland, and the muscles of mastication. Clefts of the face or lips are common. Goldenhar syndrome is considered to be part of this continuous spectrum. In addition to the underdevelopment of the components mentioned, Goldenhar syndrome is characterized by vertebral anomalies and epibulbar dermoids.

Other classifications have attempted to take into account both soft tissue and hard tissue deformities and to relate the degree of deformity to the treatment modalities available. An alphanumeric coding system, SAT, provides cohesion to existing hemifacial microsomia classifications (David et al., 1987). The acronym SAT is derived from: S = *s*keletal, A = *a*uricle, T = soft *t*issue. There are five levels of skeletal deformity (S_1–S_5), four levels of auricular deformity (A_0–A_3), and three levels of soft tissue deformity (T_1–T_3). Levels S_1–S_3 are adapted from the grades of mandibular deformity proposed by Pruzansky (1969). Patients with orbital involvement may be allocated further to levels S_4 or S_5, after Lauritzen et al. (1985). A normal auricle is represented by A_0, with A_1, A_2, and A_3 following the grades of microtia described by Meurman (1957). The soft tissue category has three levels, ranging from minimal deformity (T_1) to severe deformity (T_3), similar to the grading of Murray et al. (1984).

Skeletal categories

S_1 = Small mandible with normal shape (Figs. 5.19C–F).

S_2 = Condyle, ramus, and sigmoid notch identifiable but grossly distorted. Mandible strikingly different in size and shape from normal (Figs. 5.21C,D).

S_3 = Mandible severely malformed, ranging from poorly identifiable ramus components to complete agenesis of ramus (Figs. 5.22C–E).

S_4 = S_3 mandible plus orbital involvement with gross posterior recession of lateral and inferior orbital rims (Figs. 5.23G–I).

S_5 = S_4 defects plus orbital dystopia and frequently hypoplasia; asymmetrical neurocranium with a flat temporal fossa (Figs. 5.24C–E).

Aurical categories

A_0 = Normal.

A_1 = Small, malformed auricle retaining characteristic features (Figs. 5.23A–E).

A_2 = Rudimentary auricle with hook at cranial end corresponding to the helix.

A_3 = Malformed lobule with the rest of the pinna absent (Figs. 5.20A,B and 5.22A,B).

Soft tissue categories

T_1 = Minimal contour defect with no cranial nerve involvement (Fig. 5.19A).

T_2 = Moderate defect (Fig. 5.20A,B).

T_3 = Major defect with obvious facial scoliosis and possible severe hypoplasia of cranial nerves, parotid gland, muscles of mastication, eye involvement, and clefts of face or lips (Figs. 5.23A and 5.24A,B).

Recommended Reading

Boo-Chai K: The oblique facial cleft: a report of 2 cases and a review of 41 cases. Br J Plast Surg 23:352, 1970.

Converse JM, Wood-Smith D, McCarthy JG, et al: Bilateral facial microsomia—diagnosis, classification, treatment. Plast Reconstr Surg 54:413, 1974.

Converse JM, McCarthy JG, Coccaro PJ, Wood-Smith D: Clinical aspects of craniofacial microsomia. In Converse JM, McCarthy JG, Wood-Smith D (eds): Symposium on Diagnosis and Treatment of Craniofacial Anomalies. Mosby, St. Louis, p 461, 1979.

David DJ, Mahatumarat C, Cooter RD: Hemifacial microsomia—a multisystem classification. Plast Reconstr Surg 80:525, 1987.

DeMeyer W, Zeman W, Palmer CA: The face predicts the brain: diagnostic significance of median facial anomalies for holoprosencephaly (arhinencephaly). Pediatrics 34:256, 1964.

Dey DL: Oblique facial clefts. Plast Reconstr Surg 52:258, 1973.

Esser E: La fissure médiane du nez. Plast Chir 1:40, 1939.

Figueroa AA, Pruzansky S: The external ear, mandible and other components of hemifacial microsomia. J Maxillofac Surg 10:200, 1982.

Fogh-Anderson P: Rare clefts of the face. Acta Chir Scand 129:275, 1965.

Gosserez M, Stricker M: Dysraphies faciales médianes: le neuropore antérieur et le cerveau olfactif. Ann Chir Plast 13:264, 1968.

Grabb WC: The first and second branchial arch syndrome. Plast Reconstr Surg 36:485, 1965.

Gunter GS: Nasomaxillary clefts. Plast Reconstr Surg 32:637, 1963.

Kaban LB, Mulliken JB, Murray JE: Three-dimensional approach to analysis and treatment of hemifacial microsomia. Cleft Palate J 18:90, 1981.

Karfik V: Proposed classification of rare congenital cleft malformations in the face. Acta Chir Plast 8:163, 1966.

Kawamoto HK: The kaleidoscopic world of rare craniofacial clefts: order out of chaos (Tessier classification). Clin Plast Surg 3:529, 1976.

Lauritzen C, Munro IR, Ross RB: Classification and treatment of hemifacial microsomia. Scand J Plast Reconstr Surg 19:33, 1985.

Mazzola RF: Congenital malformations in the frontonasal area: their pathogenesis and classification. Clin Plast Surg 3:573, 1976.

McKenzie J, Craig J: Mandibulo-facial dysostosis (Treacher Collins syndrome). Arch Dis Child 30:391, 1955.

Meurman Y: Congenital microtia and meatal atresia. AMA Arch Otolaryngol 66:443, 1957.

Millard DR: Cleft Craft: The Evolution of Its Surgery. Vols 1–3. Little, Brown, Boston, 1976.

Morian R: Über die schräge Gesichtsspalte. Arch Klin Chir 35:245, 1887.

Murray JE, Kaban LB, Mulliken JB: Analysis and treatment of hemifacial microsomia. Plast Reconstr Surg 74:186, 1984.

Pfeifer G: Systematik und Morphologie der kraniofazialen Anomalien. Fortschr Kiefer Gesichtschir 18:1, 1974.

Poswillo D: The pathogenesis of Treacher Collins syndrome (mandibulo-facial dysostosis). Br J Oral Surg 13:1, 1975.

Pruzansky S: Not all dwarfed mandibles are alike. Birth Defects 5:120, 1969.

Raulo Y, Tessier P: Mandibulo-facial dysostosis analysis: principles of surgery. Scand J Plast Reconstr Surg 15:251, 1981.

Rogers BO: Rare craniofacial deformities. In Converse JM (ed): Reconstructive Plastic Surgery. Vol 3. Saunders, Philadelphia, p 1213, 1964.

Sanvenero-Rosselli G: Developmental pathology of the face and the dysraphic syndrome—an essay of interpretation based on experimentally produced congenital defects. Plast Reconstr Surg 11:36, 1953.

Swanson LT, Murray JE: Asymmetries of the lower part of the face. In Whitaker LA, Randall P (eds): Symposium on Reconstruction of Jaw Deformity. Vol 16. Mosby, St. Louis, p 171, 1978.

Tessier P: Anatomical classification of facial, craniofacial, and laterofacial clefts. J Maxillofac Surg 4:69, 1976.

Van der Meulen JCH: Obique facial clefts: pathology, etiology, and reconstruction. Plast Reconstr Surg 76:212, 1985.

A B

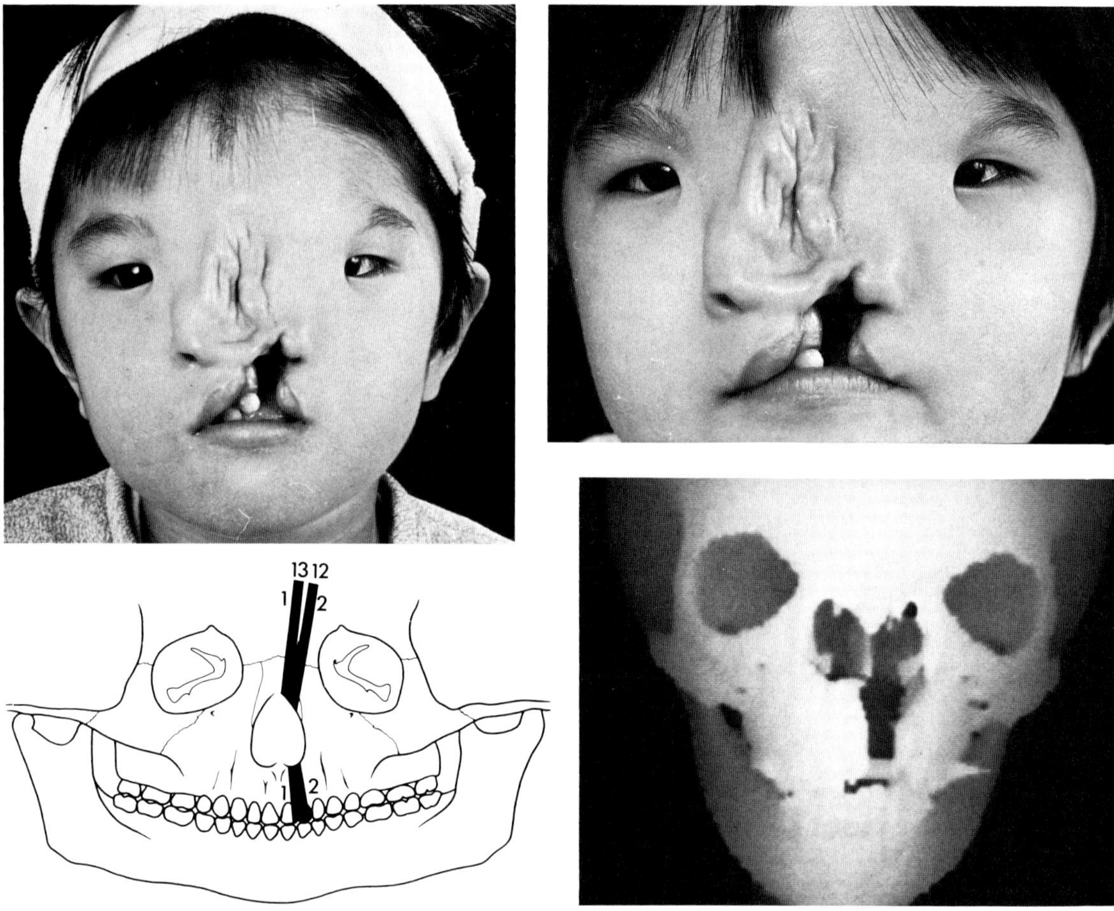

C D

E

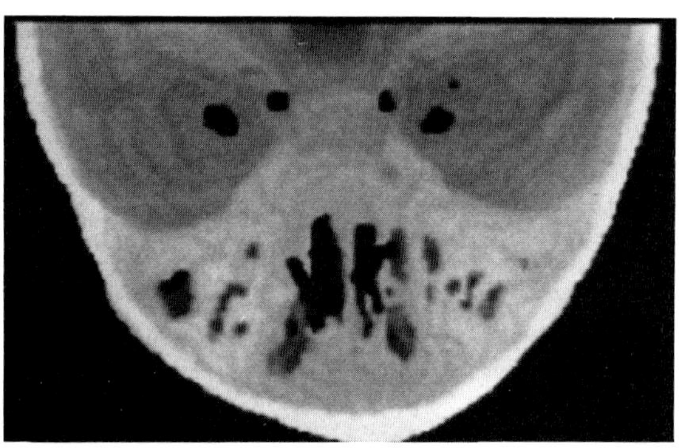

Fig. 5.1. A Complex paramedian clefts have produced gross hypertelorism. There is left-sided clefting of the lip and palate. Distorted nasal elements are associated with a deranged maxilla. **B** Wrinkling of nasal skin is a rare deformity. **C** Tessier cleft numbering of patient in Figure 5.1A. **D** Wide interorbital distance is apparent on the three-dimensional image, which also shows the cleft extending down through the maxilla. **E** Anterior fossa view is often helpful for assessing the deeper distortion caused by a cleft.

A

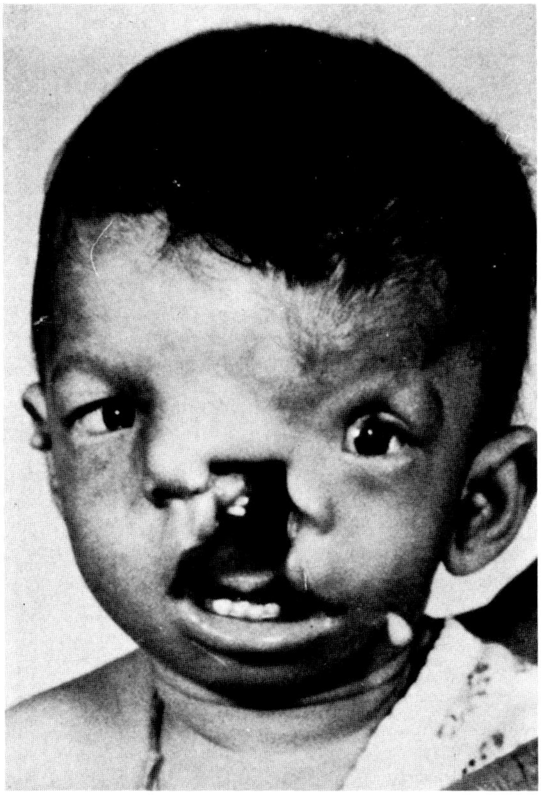

C

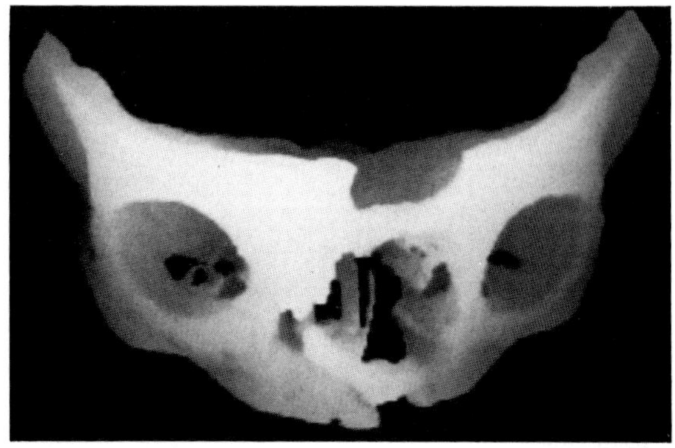

D

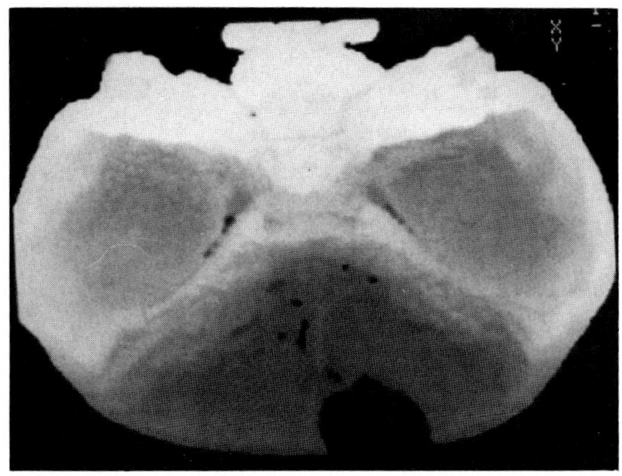

B

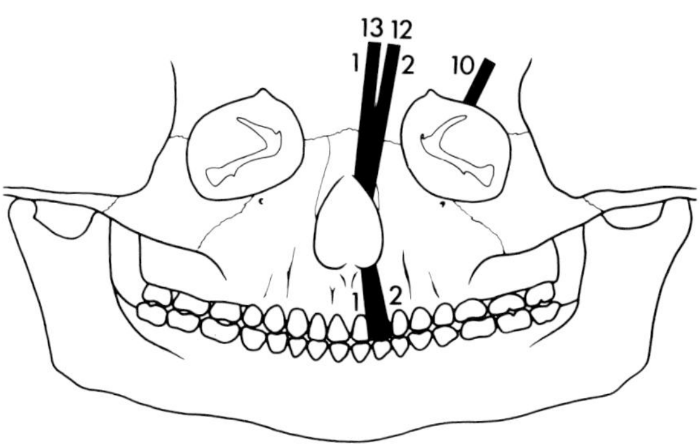

Fig. 5.2. A Wide central cleft has produced hypertelorism. Additionally, there is a cleft extending laterally from the region of the left brow. **B** Tessier cleft numbering of patient in Figure 5.2A. **C** The left eye is further displaced from the midline than the right eye. The frontal cleft extends into the maxilla with subsequent distortion of the premaxilla. **D** In the basal view the cleft can be seen to involve the anterior cranial fossa, whereas the middle cranial fossae are not affected.

A

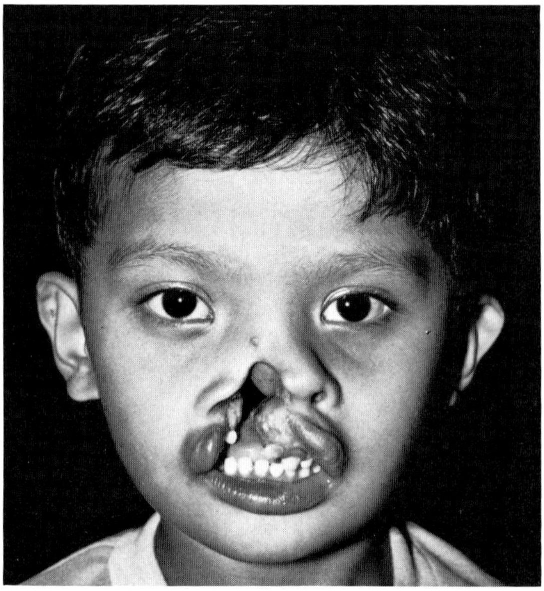

C

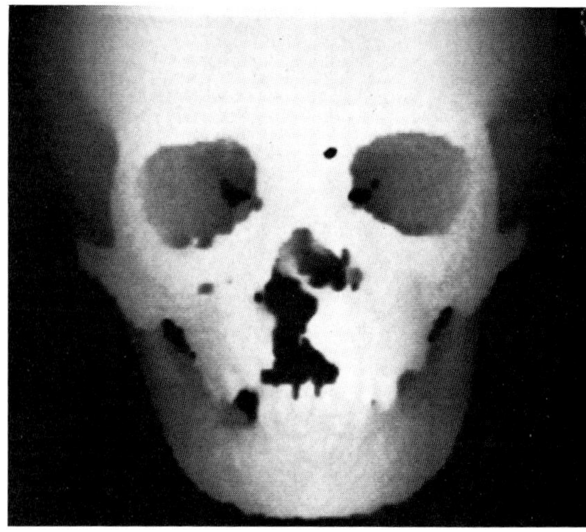

B

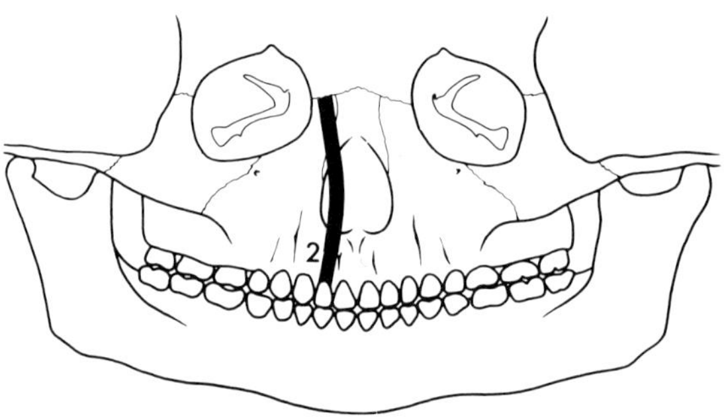

Fig. 5.3. A This No. 2 cleft, located on the right, involves the lip and palate. It extends through the alveolus upward through the dome of the right nostril. The medial canthus is widened on the right. **B** Tessier cleft numbering of patient in Figure 5.3A. **C** Absence of central support for the maxillary arch has resulted in medial collapse of the alveolar segments.

A

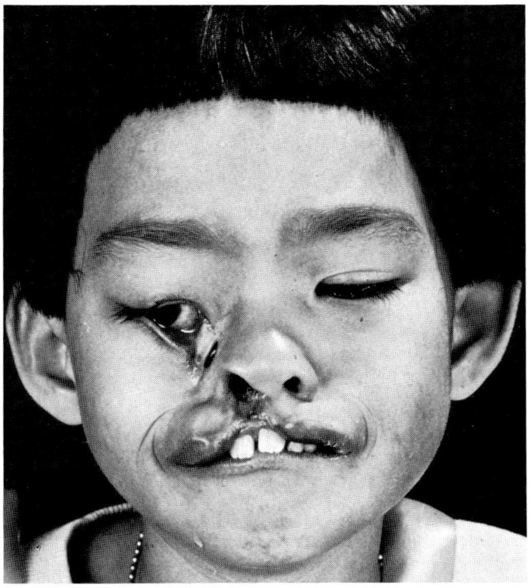

B

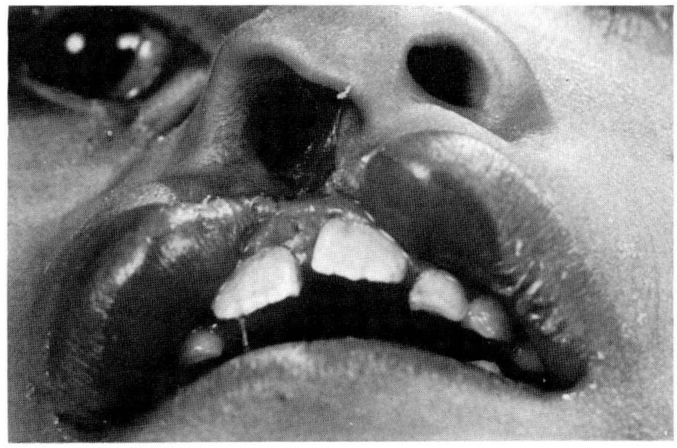

C

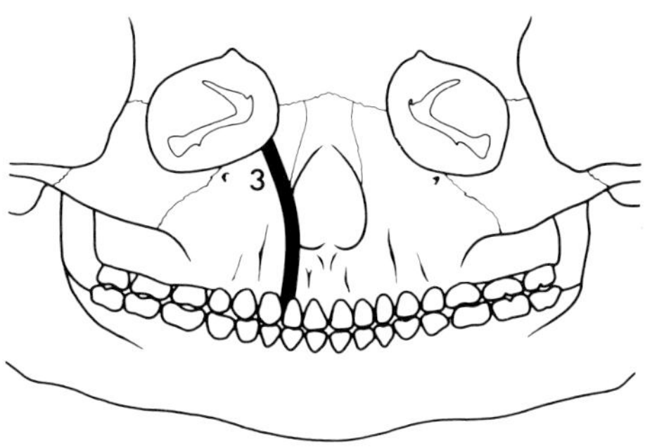

D

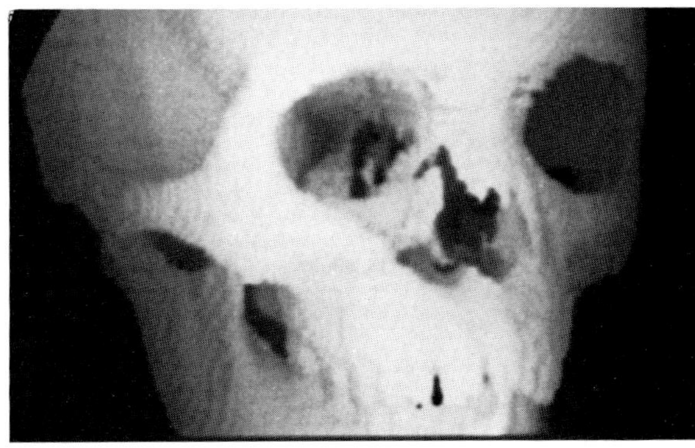

Fig. 5.4. A,B Cleft passes through the upper lip and involves the lateral aspect of the right nostril. It then extends into the region of the lacrimal apparatus, producing a coloboma of the lower eyelid and lowering of the globe on that side. **C** Tessier cleft numbering of patient in Figure 5.4A. **D** There is bony deficiency of the nasal bone and the lateral wall of the nose in the region of the lacrimal apparatus.

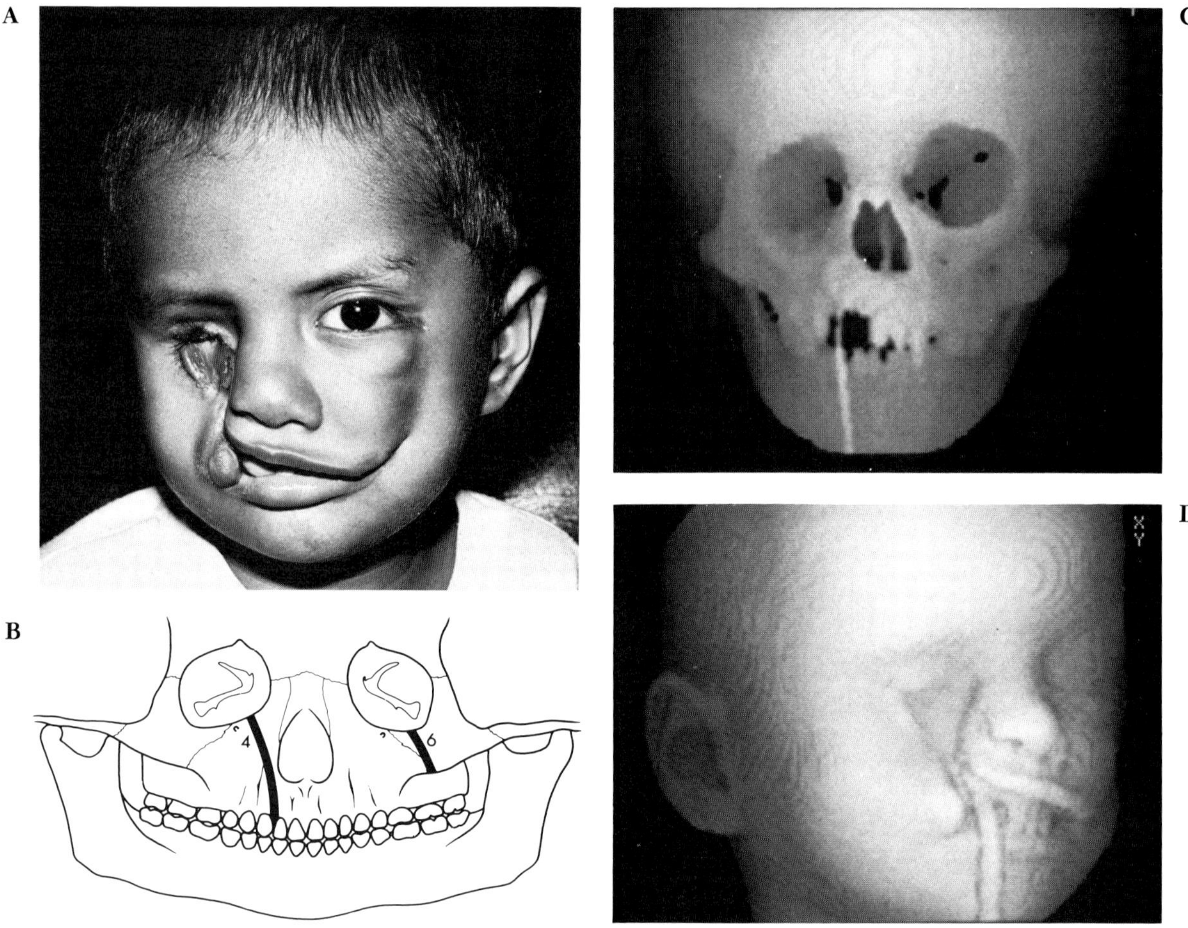

Fig. 5.5. A Right-sided No. 4 cleft and left-sided No. 6 cleft with macrostomia. The right-sided cleft passes through the lower eyelid lateral to the lacrimal punctum ending in an anophthalmic orbit. **B** Tessier cleft numbering of patient in Figure 5.5A. **C** Clefting is seen passing through the alveolus and extending to a depressed infraorbital margin. It contributes to the maxillary hypoplasia on the right. **D** Soft tissue reconstructions can be made and related to the underlying hard tissue deformity based on CT scan data.

A

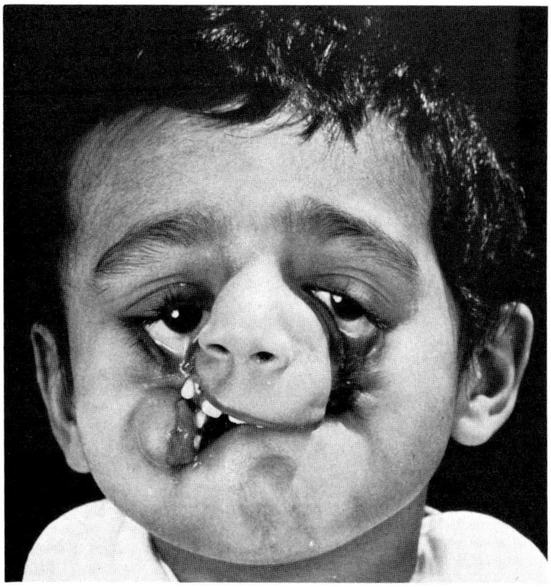

B

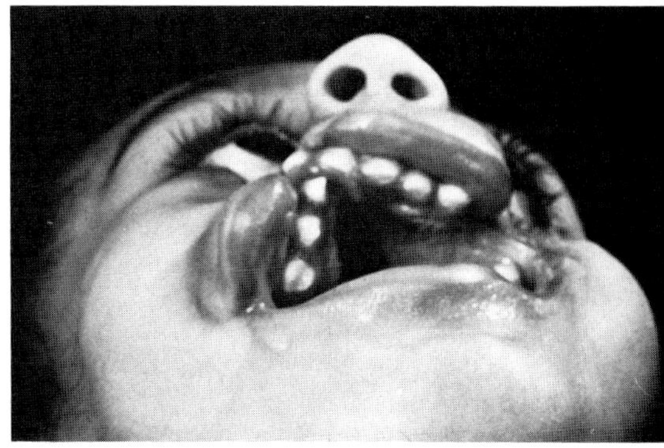

C

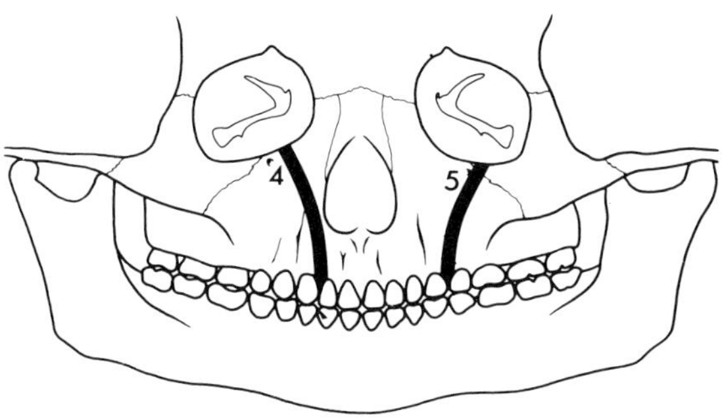

D

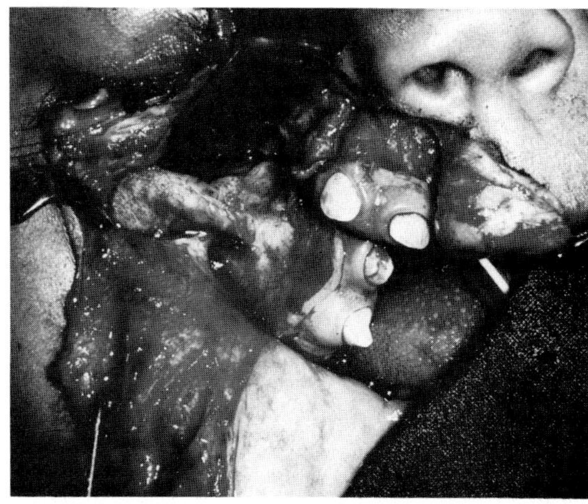

E

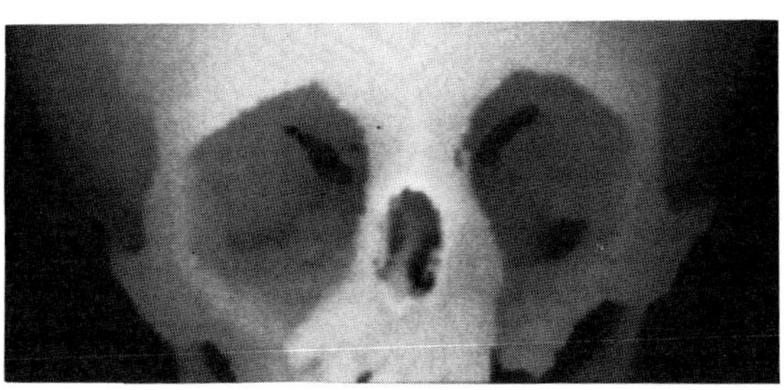

F

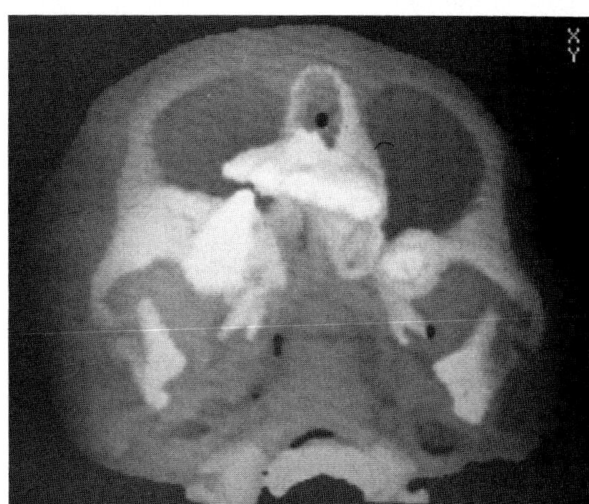

Fig. 5.6. A Severe disruption of both soft and hard tissue is typical of the paramedian clefts. **B** Bilateral facial clefts extend through the palate on the right side between the lateral incisor and the canine, and on the left side posterior to the canine. **C** Tessier cleft numbering of patient in Figure 5.6A. **D** Intraoperative view shows the No. 4 cleft passing medial to the infraorbital nerve (arrow). **E** Orbits are funnel-shaped and extend down through the maxilla. **F** There is a Tessier No. 5 cleft on the left and a Tessier No. 4 cleft on the right (confirmed at operation). The twist of the central segment and its relation to the two lateral segments of the alveolar arch are well demonstrated below the distorted orbits. Note the position of the pterygoid plates, with the right pair being more medially placed.

A

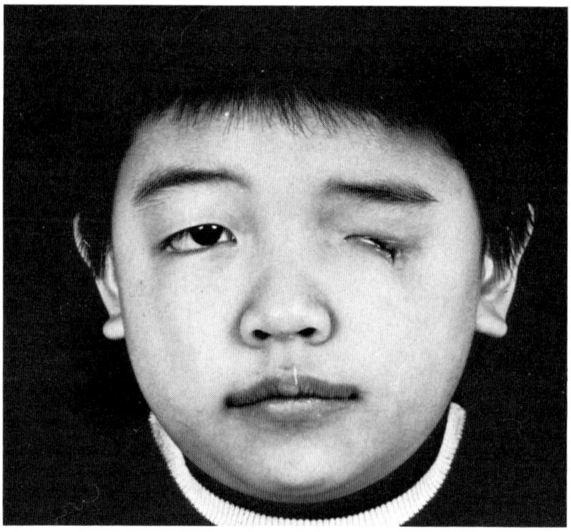

B

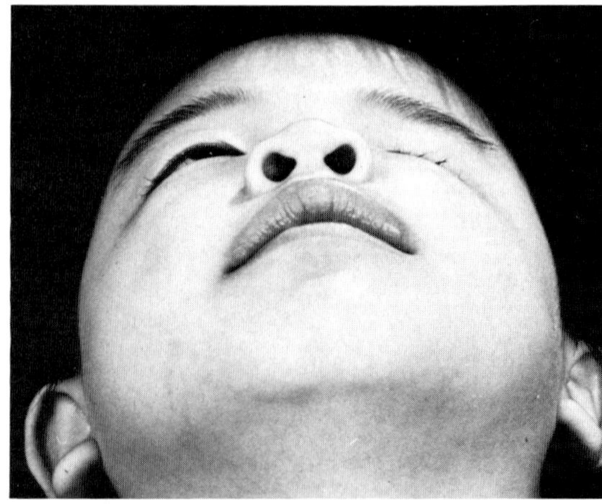

C

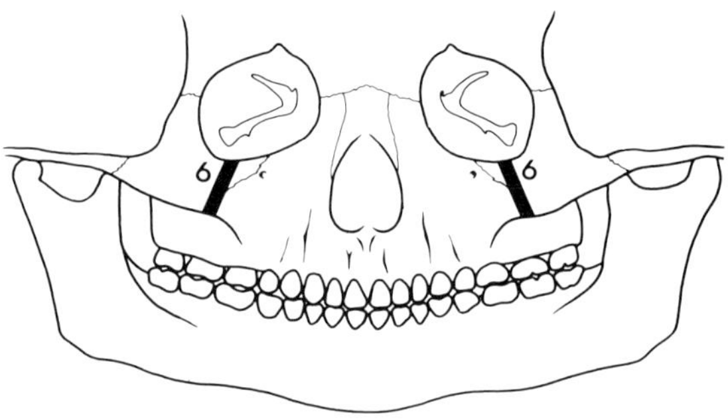

D

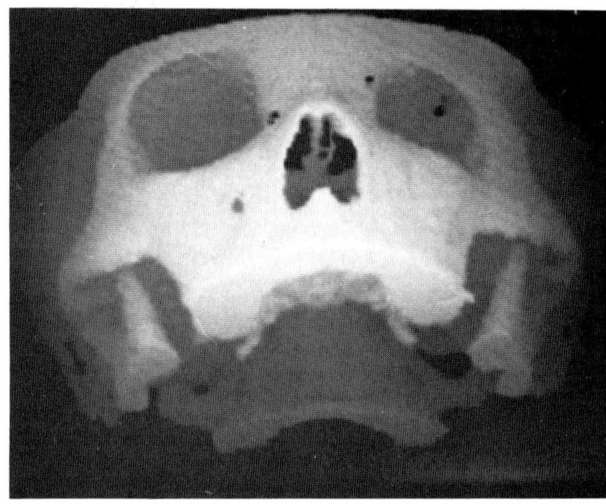

E

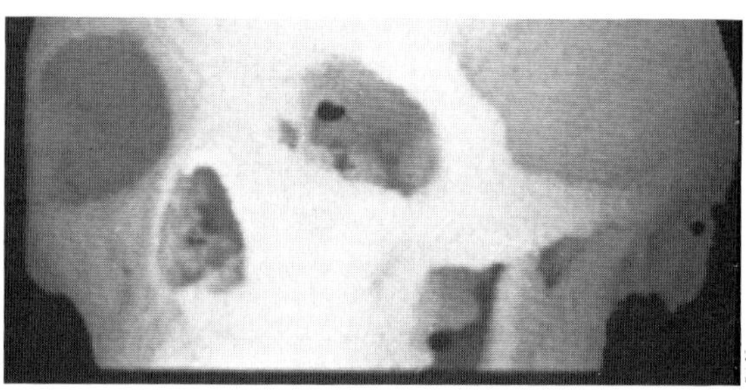

Fig. 5.7. A,B Bilateral Tessier No. 6 clefts (not Treacher Collins syndrome) and microphthalmia. Clefts originate from the region of the lateral commissure of the mouth and pass into the lateral part of the lower eyelids. Patient has normal pinnas and a symmetrical mandible. **C** Tessier cleft numbering of patient in Figure 5.7A. **D** Paramedian structures are normal, and there is no condylar hypoplasia. **E** There is a groove between the maxilla and the zygoma, more prominent on the left and associated with left orbital hypoplasia.

A C D B

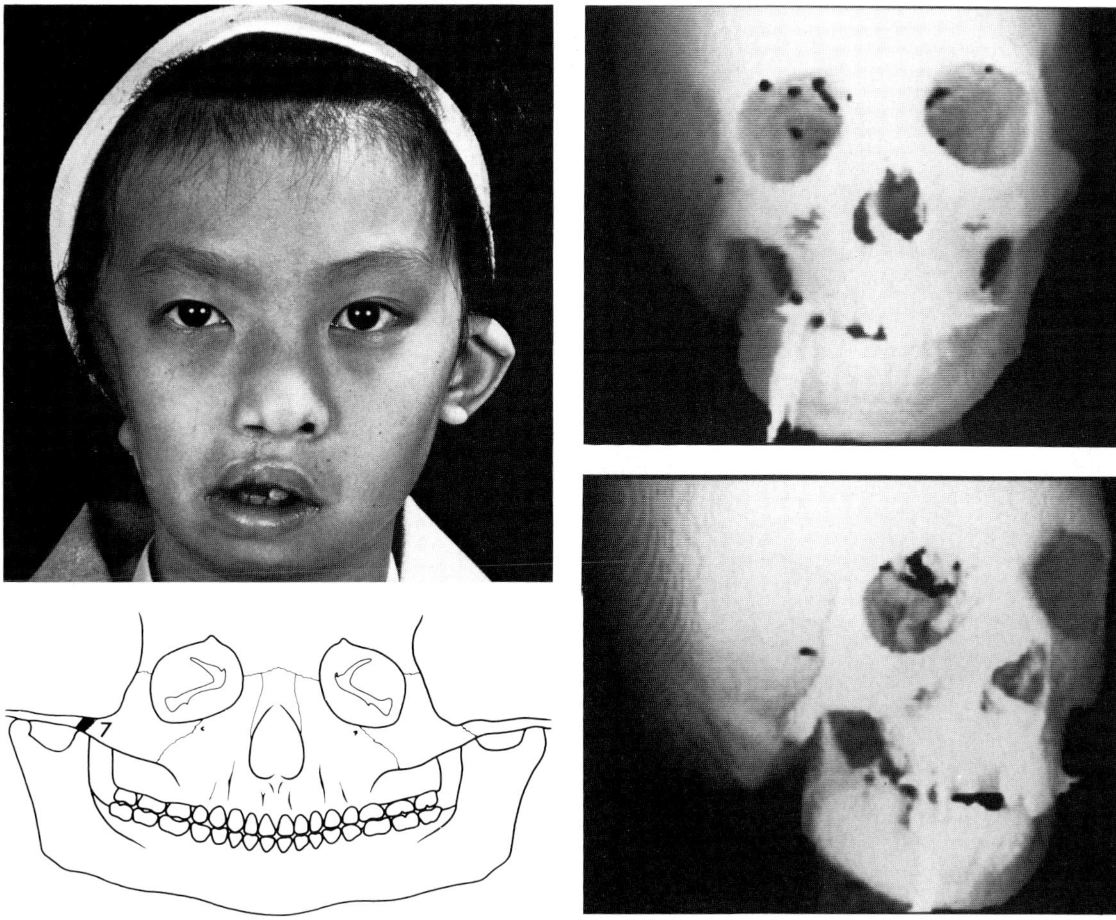

Fig. 5.8. **A** Right-sided hemifacial microsomia with macrostomia, absence of the zygomatic arch, hypoplasia of the mandible, and right anotia. **B** Tessier cleft numbering of patient in Figure 5.8A. **C** There is vertical "compression" of right-sided structures. **D** There is no right temporomandibular joint, and the right mandibular ramus is reduced to a thin, bony spur. (See also Figs. 5.19–5.24.)

A C

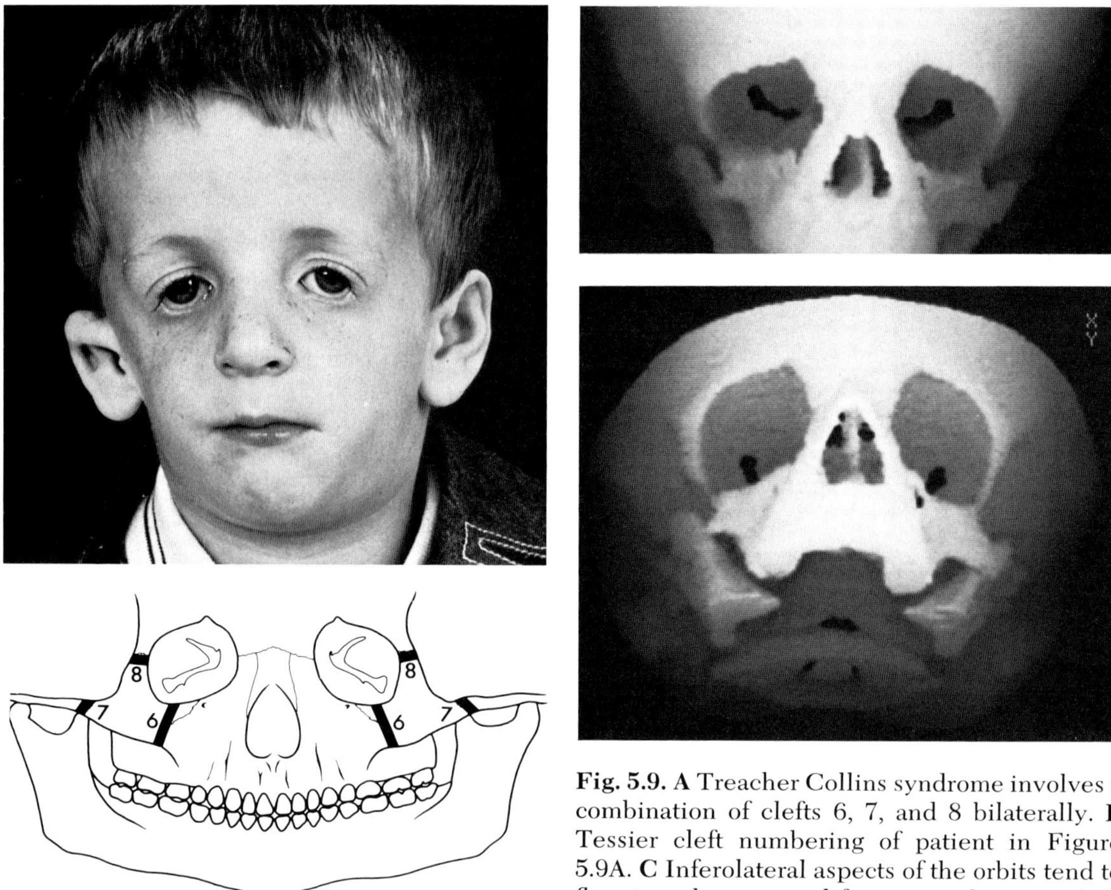

B D

Fig. 5.9. A Treacher Collins syndrome involves a combination of clefts 6, 7, and 8 bilaterally. **B** Tessier cleft numbering of patient in Figure 5.9A. **C** Inferolateral aspects of the orbits tend to flow into the temporal fossae. **D** There are deficiencies in the lateral orbital wall and zygomatic arches, and there is clefting between the zygoma and maxilla. (See also Figs. 5.16–5.18.)

A

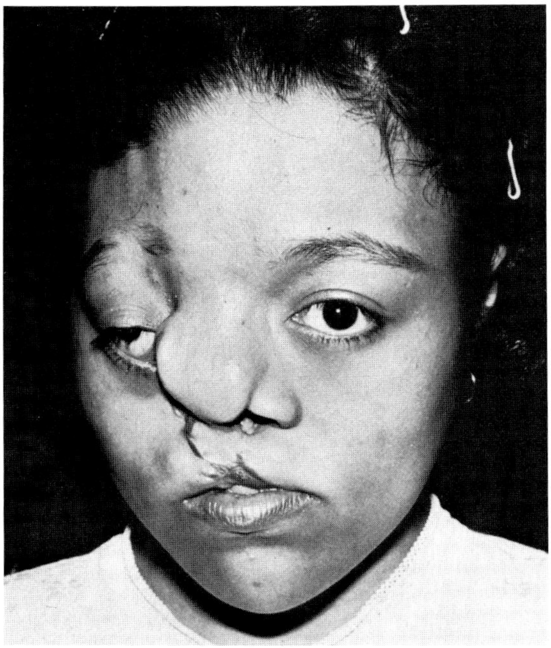

B

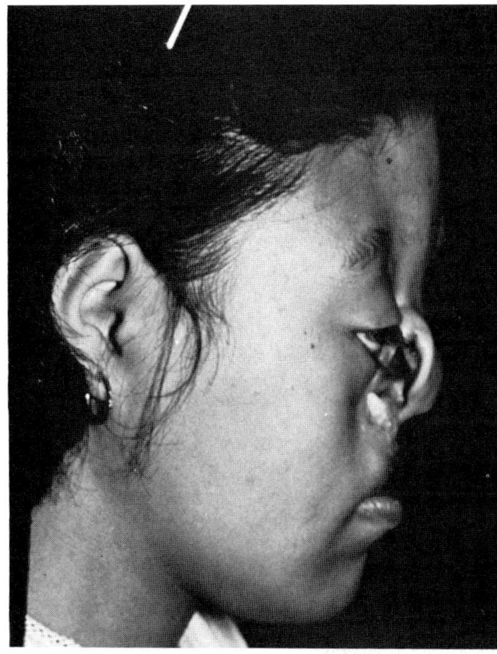

C

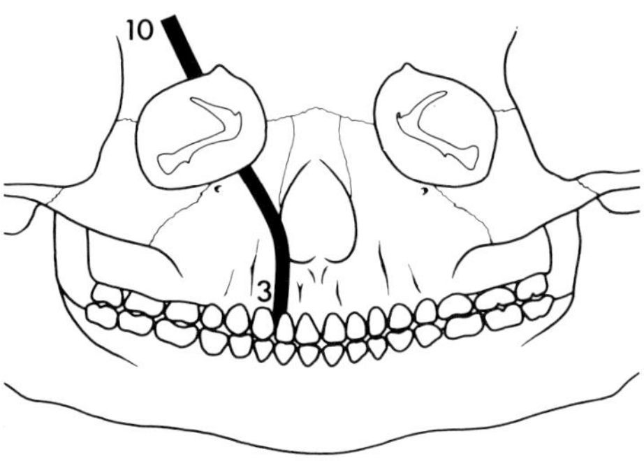

D

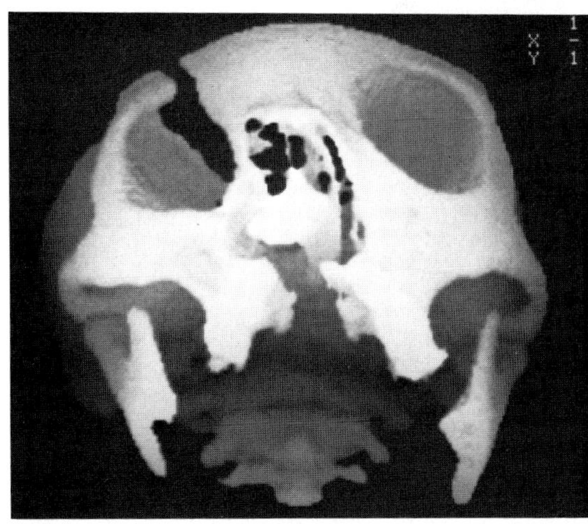

E

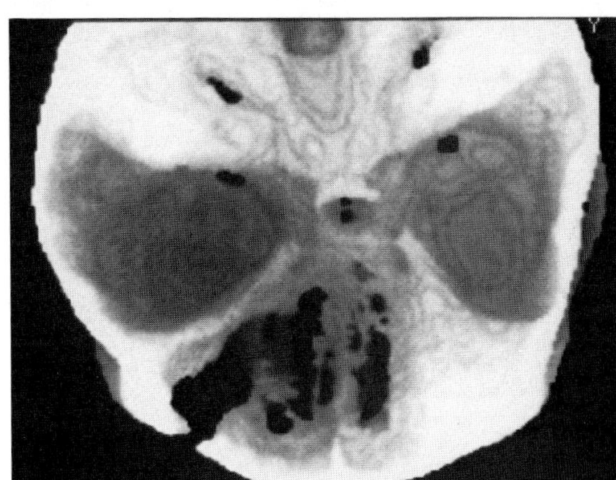

Fig. 5.10. A,B Multiple clefts affecting the right supraorbital margin, right lower eyelid, and nostril in association with bilateral cleft lip and palate. **C** Tessier cleft numbering of patient in Figure 5.10A,B. **D** Cleft of the palate with distortion of the premaxilla. There is an extension of clefting through the lateral nasal wall and the superior orbital margin. **E** Anterior cranial fossa view shows the cleft traversing the anterior cranial fossa from the superior orbital margin into the posterior aspect of the cribriform plate.

A
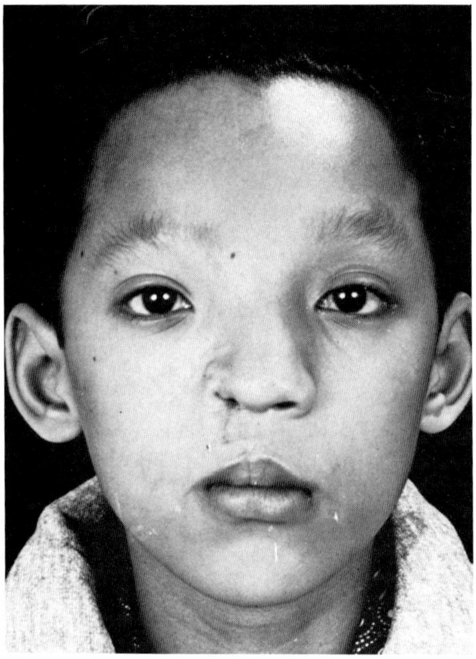

B
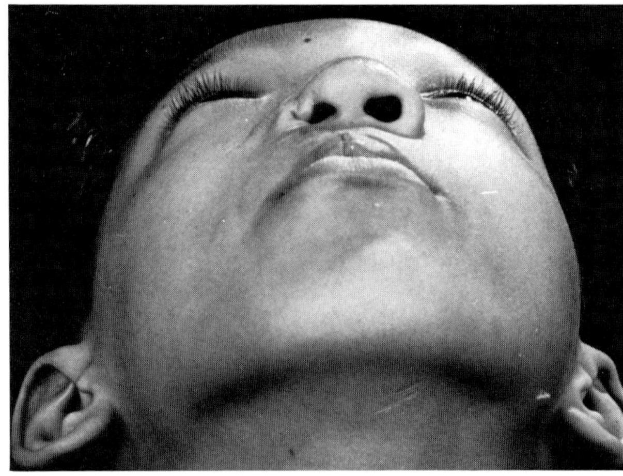

C
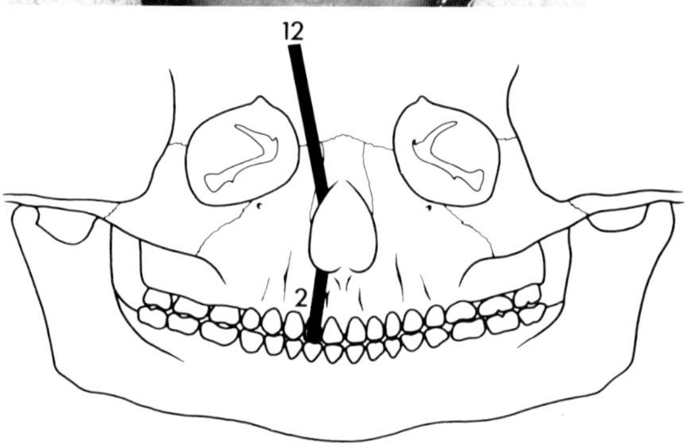

D
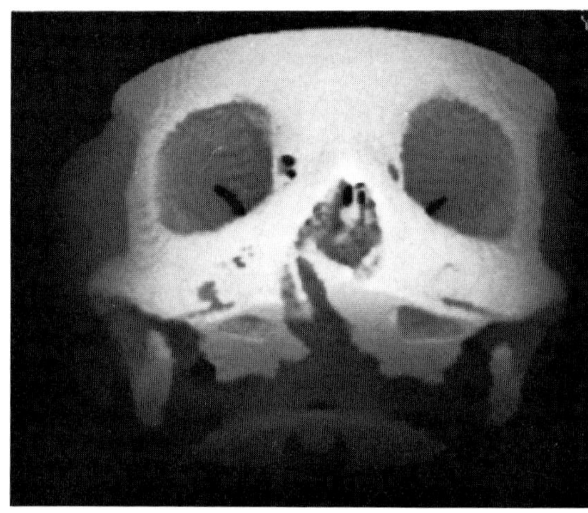

E
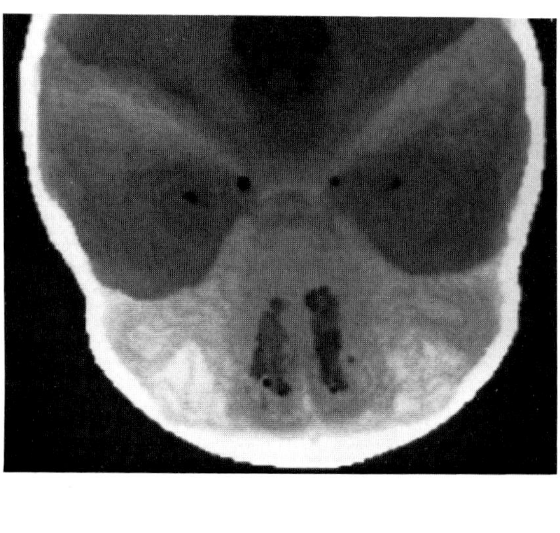

Fig. 5.11. A Upward extension of a Tessier Nos. 2/12 cleft complex has displaced this patient's right eye laterally. **B** Repaired right cleft lip with disruption of the right nostril and right-sided hypertelorism. **C** Tessier cleft numbering of patient in Figure 5.12A. **D** There is widening of the right medial canthal area as a result of the No. 12 cleft. Maxillary and palatal clefts are seen inferiorly and represent the No. 2 component. **E** Cribriform plate is widened on the right, and the anterior fossa is asymmetrical. This configuration reflects the uppermost bony distortion of the No. 12 cleft in this patient.

A

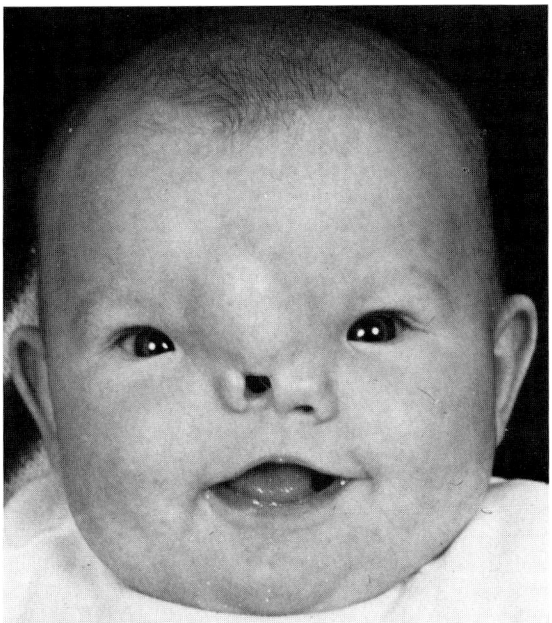

C

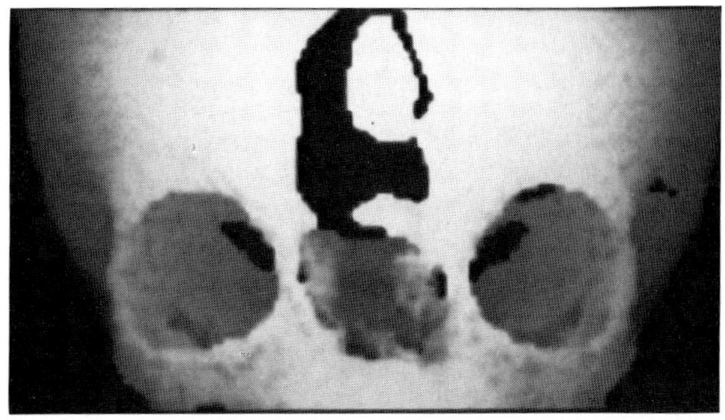

D

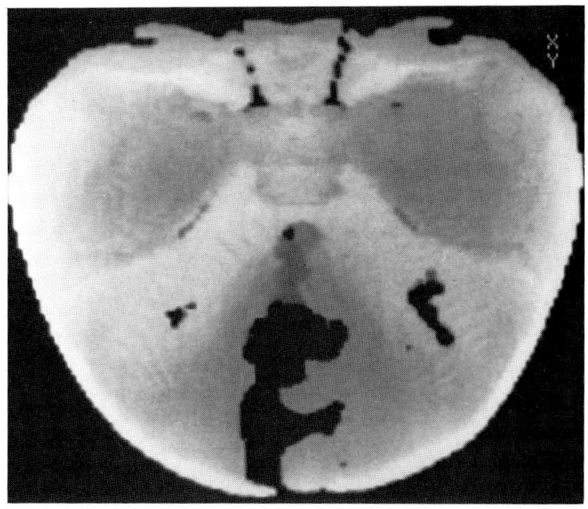

B

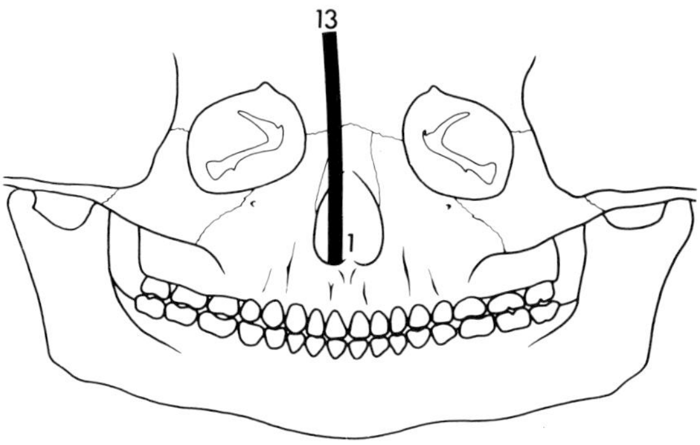

Fig. 5.12. A Cleft through the dome of the right nostril is associated with a subcutaneous lipoma and hypertelorism. **B** Tessier cleft numbering of patient in Figure 5.12A. **C** Asymmetrical clefting produced hypertelorism, wider on the right. **D** Cleft enters the right side of the cribriform plate.

A B C D E

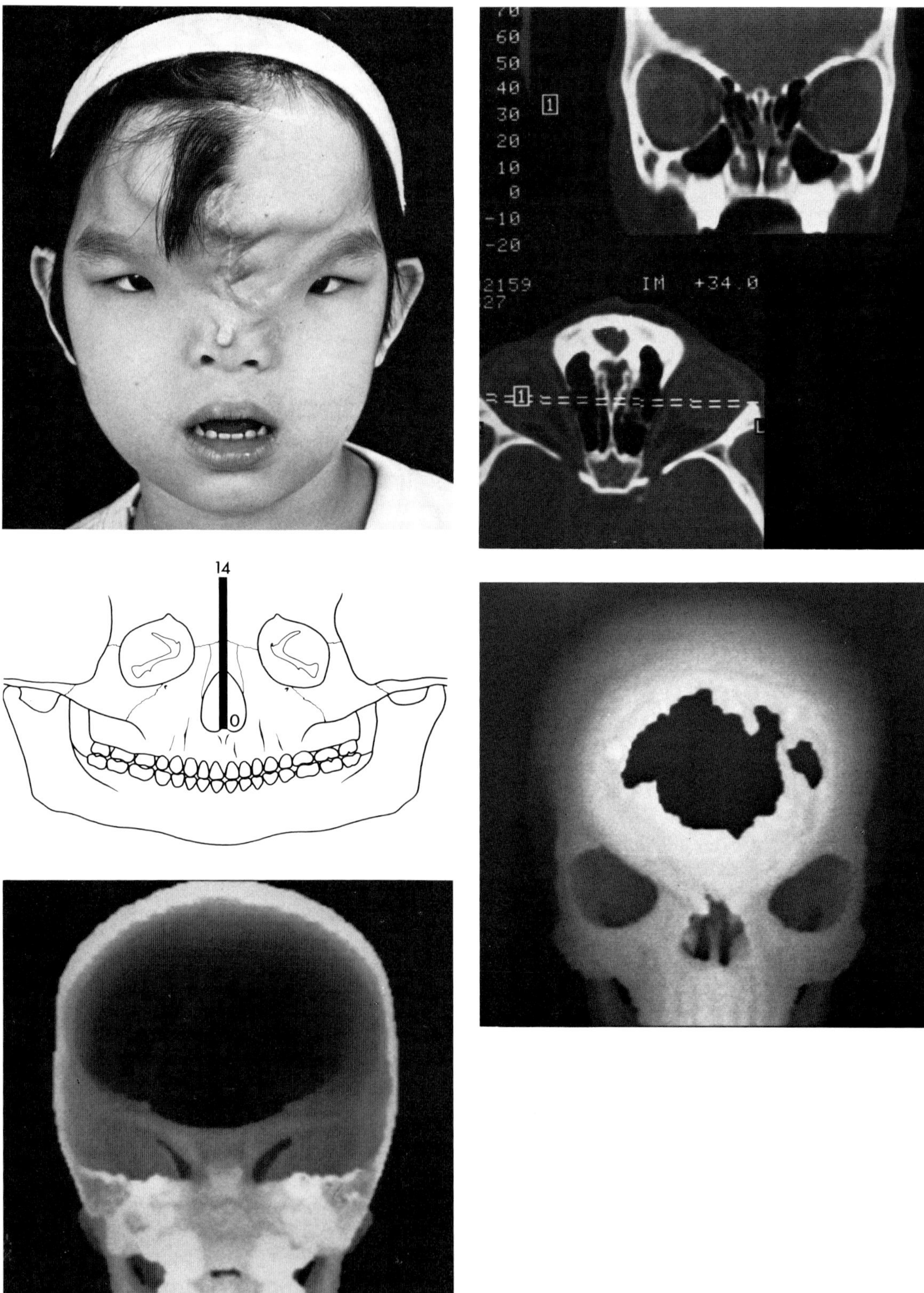

A

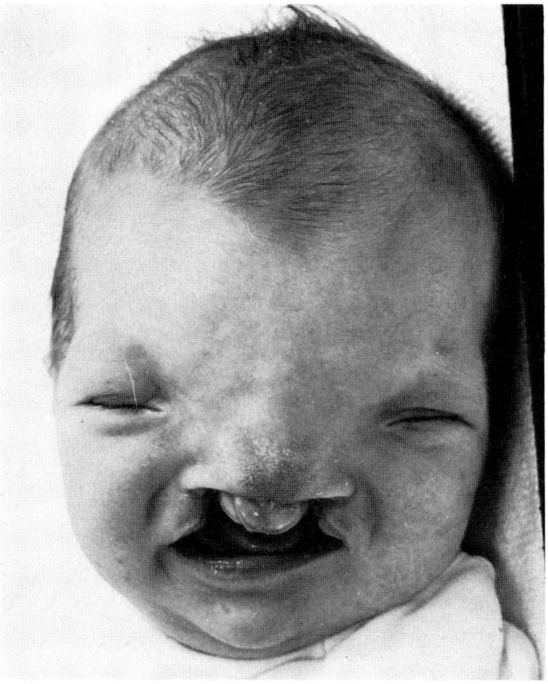

C

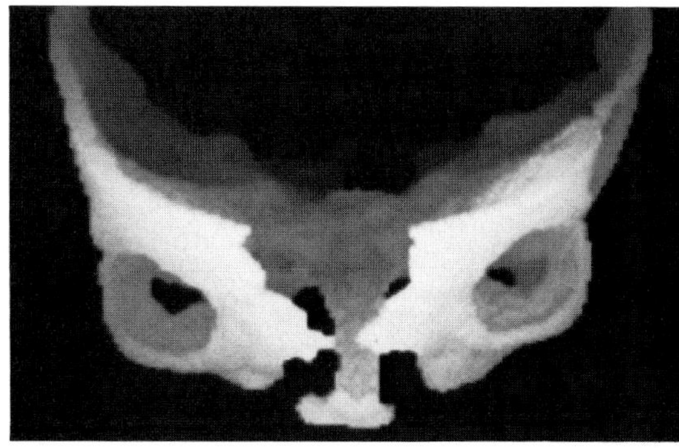

D

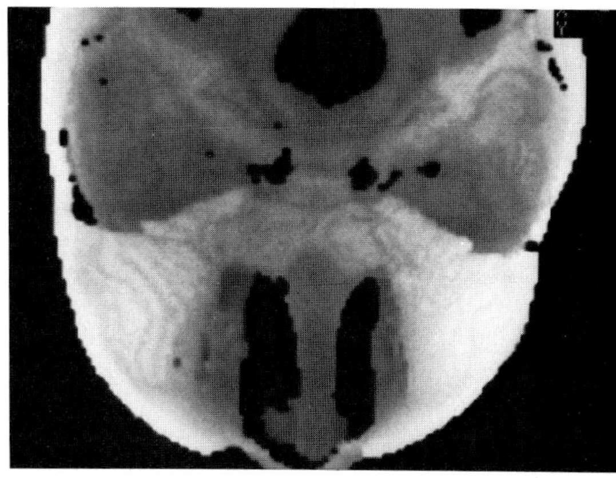

B

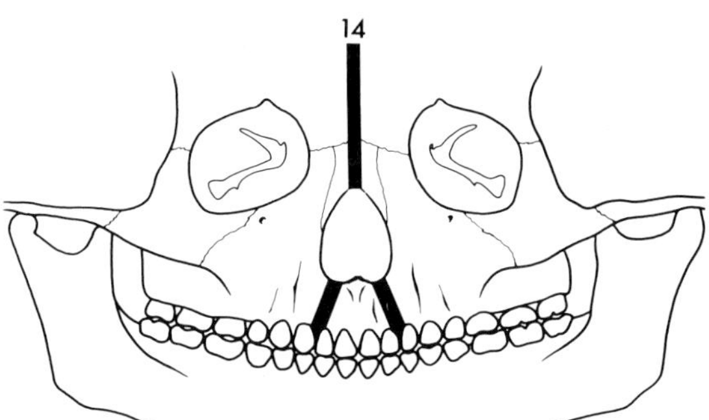

Fig. 5.14. A Midline cleft associated with bilateral cleft lip and palate. **B** Tessier cleft numbering of patient in Figure 5.14A. **C** Gross hypertelorism secondary to clefting. **D** Anterior fossa is asymmetrical. The cleft enters the anterior aspect of the cribriform plate, which is depressed and widened.

Fig. 5.13. A Midline clefting has produced gross hypertelorism. Midline tongue of hair projects down over a central encephalocele. **B** Tessier cleft numbering of patient in Figure 5.13A. **C** The degree of hypertelorism is displayed on coronal section. The greater wing of the sphenoid is rotated outward, and there is an increased mass of tissue between the medial orbital walls. **D** There is a central bony deformity in the frontal region through which an encephalocele herniates. **E** From the middle fossa the central defect in the frontal bone can be viewed from behind. There is broadening of the central structures of the anterior fossa. Note the optic foramina and superior orbital fissures.

A

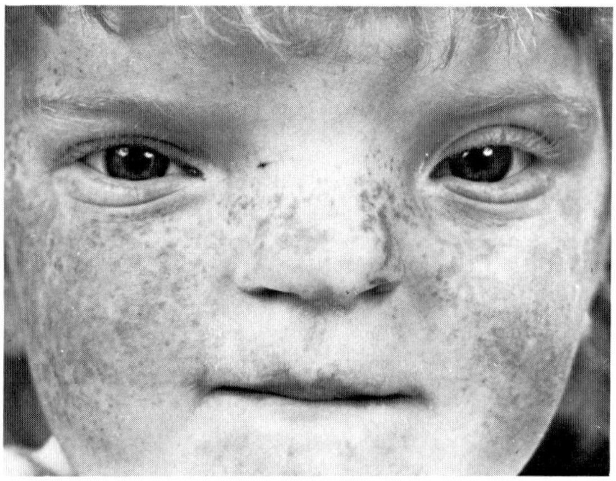

B

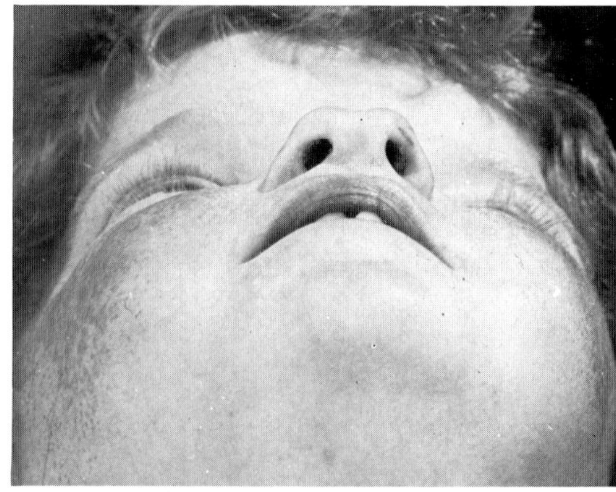

C

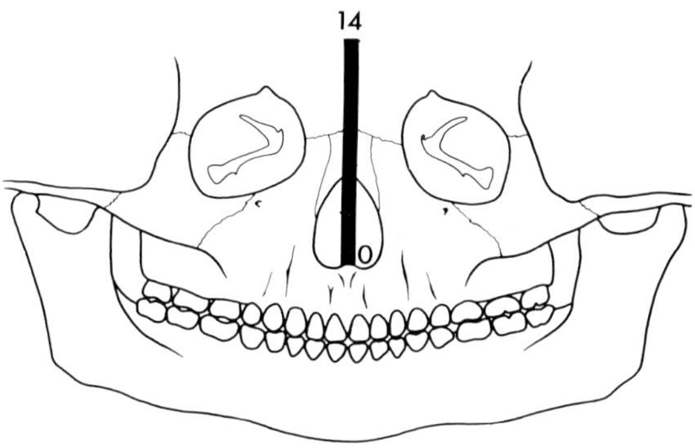

D

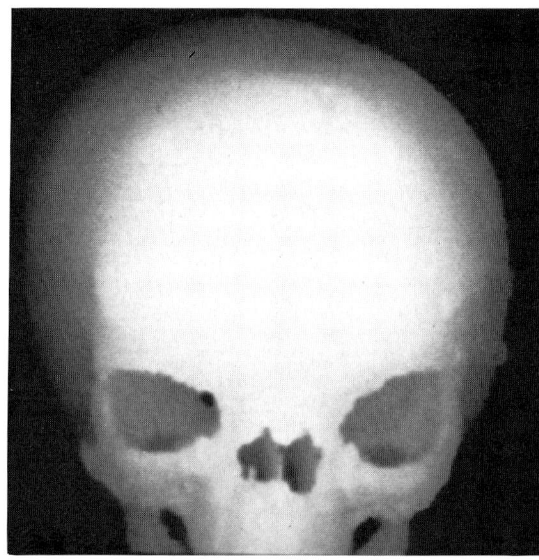

E

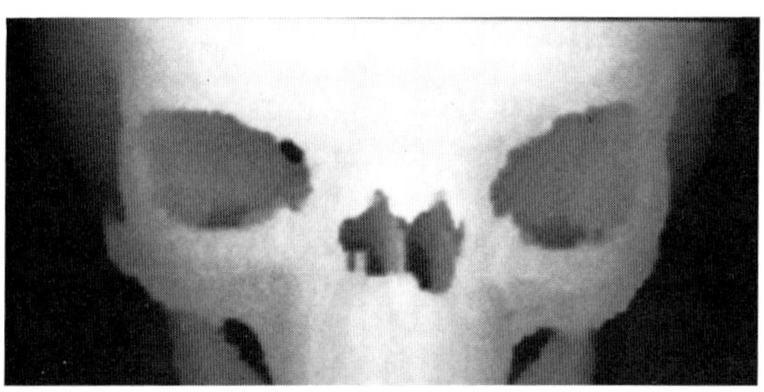

F

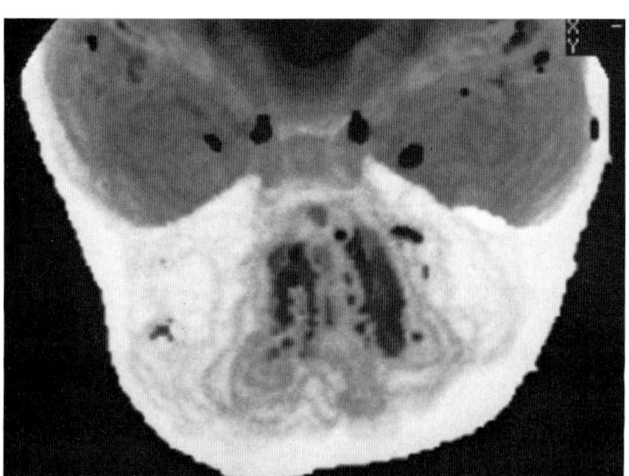

Fig. 5.15. A,B Hypertelorism secondary to a midline cleft associated with a bifid nose and a degree of frontal plagiocephaly (Cohen syndrome). **C** Tessier cleft numbering of patient in Figure 5.15A,B. **D,E** Three-dimensional reconstructions show a midline cranial type 0 cleft with an asymmetrical skull and hypertelorism. **F** Asymmetry of the anterior fossa is associated with a recessed left forehead. It has resulted from left frontal plagiocephaly.

A B C D

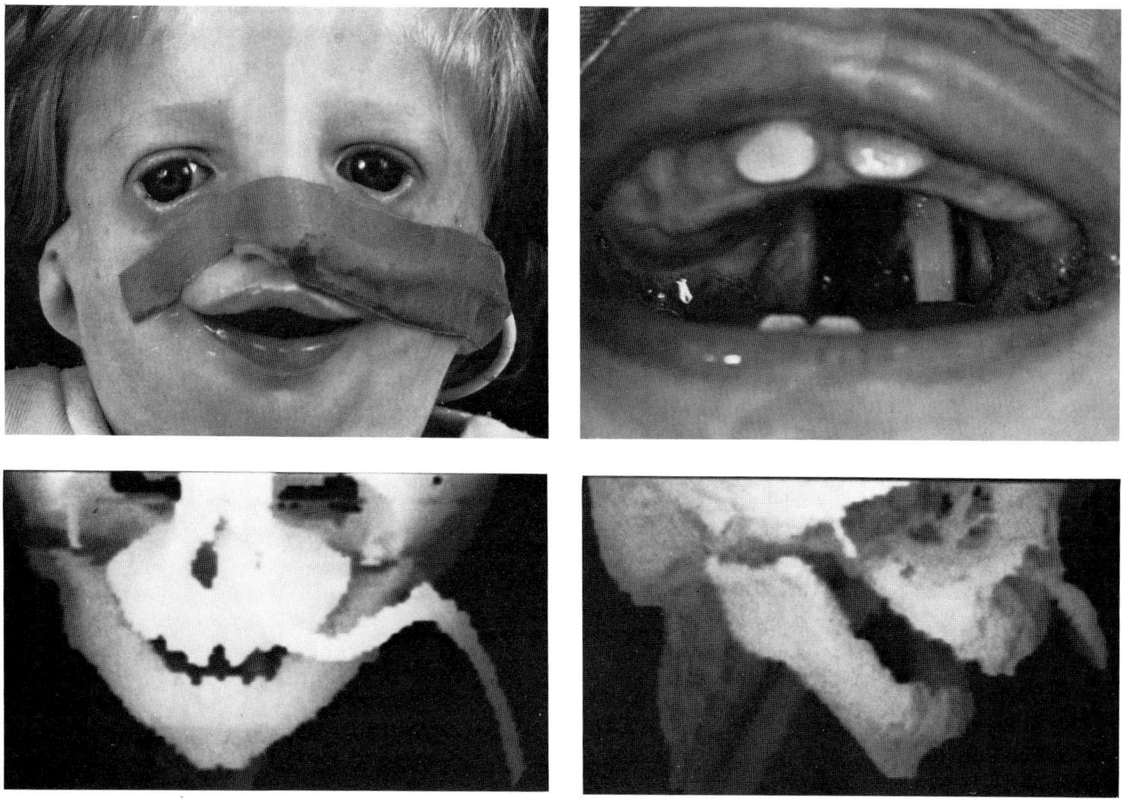

E

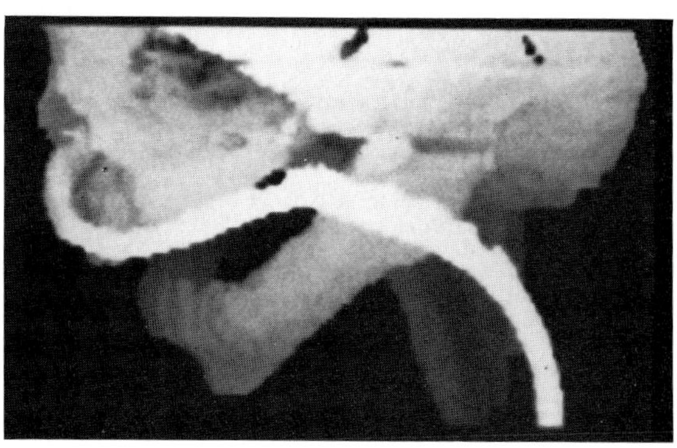

Fig. 5.16. A Severe Treacher Collins syndrome with nasal intubation. Note the bilateral macrostomia, severe ear deformities, lower eyelid colobomata, and a small mandible. **B** Intraoral view demonstrates a cleft palate. **C** Severe clefting in this syndrome produces gross deformities in the inferolateral aspects of the orbits. **D,E** Right and left osseous images demonstrate the severe deformity of the mandible, absence of the zygomatic arches, and connection between the orbit and the infratemporal fossa.

A

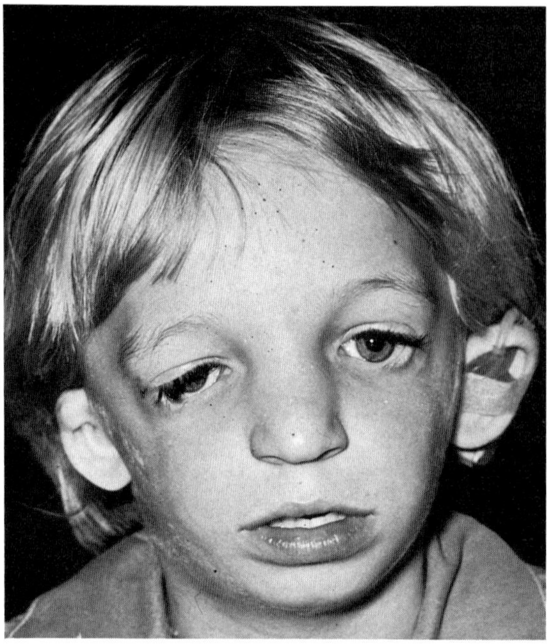

B

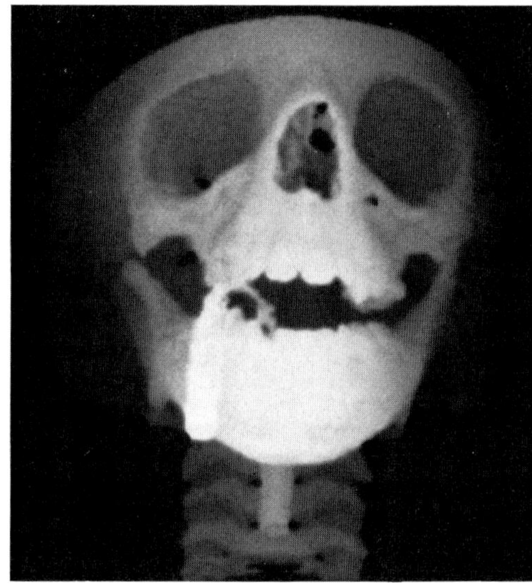

C

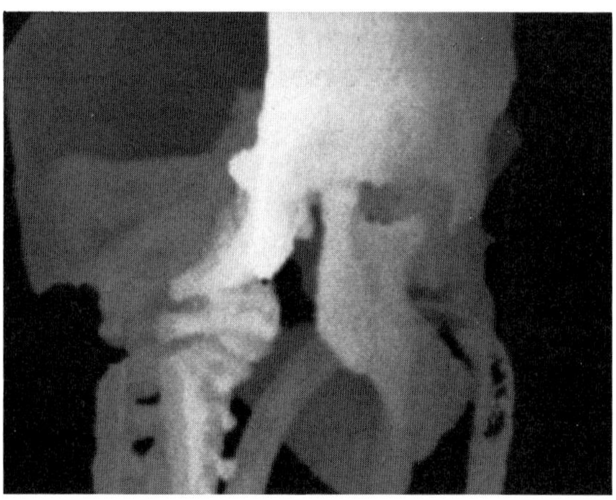

Fig. 5.17. A Example of the asymmetrical nature of Treacher Collins deformities, which are worse on the right. **B** The underlying bony abnormalities include hypoplasia of the zygomatic arch, which is worse on the right. **C** Posterior oblique view from the right side shows the flattened condylar process, lower border notch, and typical distortion of the mandible with a flattened, retrodisplaced chin.

Fig. 5.18. A Typical facies of an adult with Treacher Collins syndrome. **B** A tongue of hair is found extending onto the cheek. **C,D** Right and left lateral views indicate the relatively mild orbital deformity in this patient but absent zygomatic arches and distortion of the temporomandibular joints. There is typical lower border notching of the mandible and characteristic chin retrodisplacement. **E** Patient's family photograph indicates the dominant genetic nature of this condition. ▶

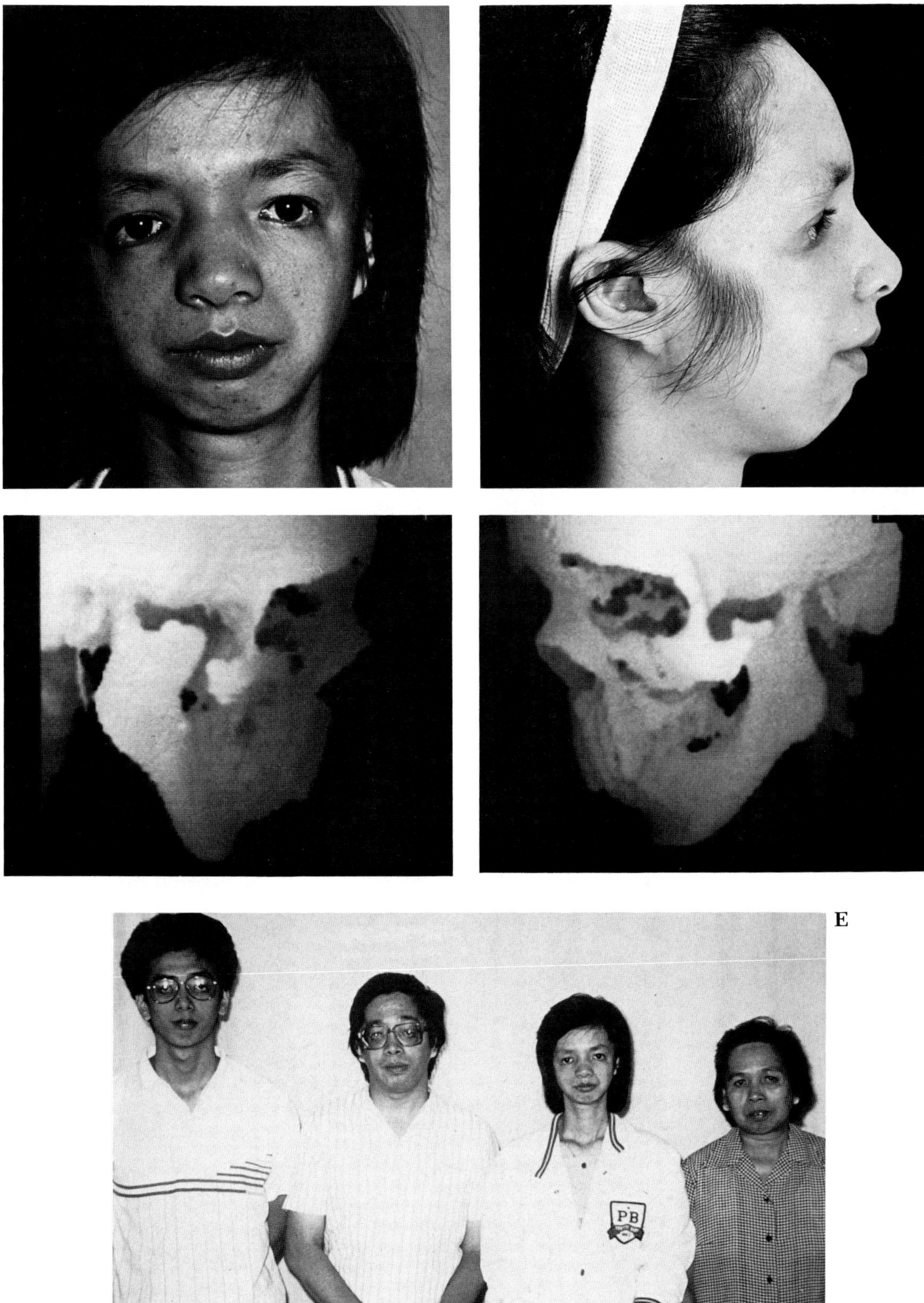
A B C D E

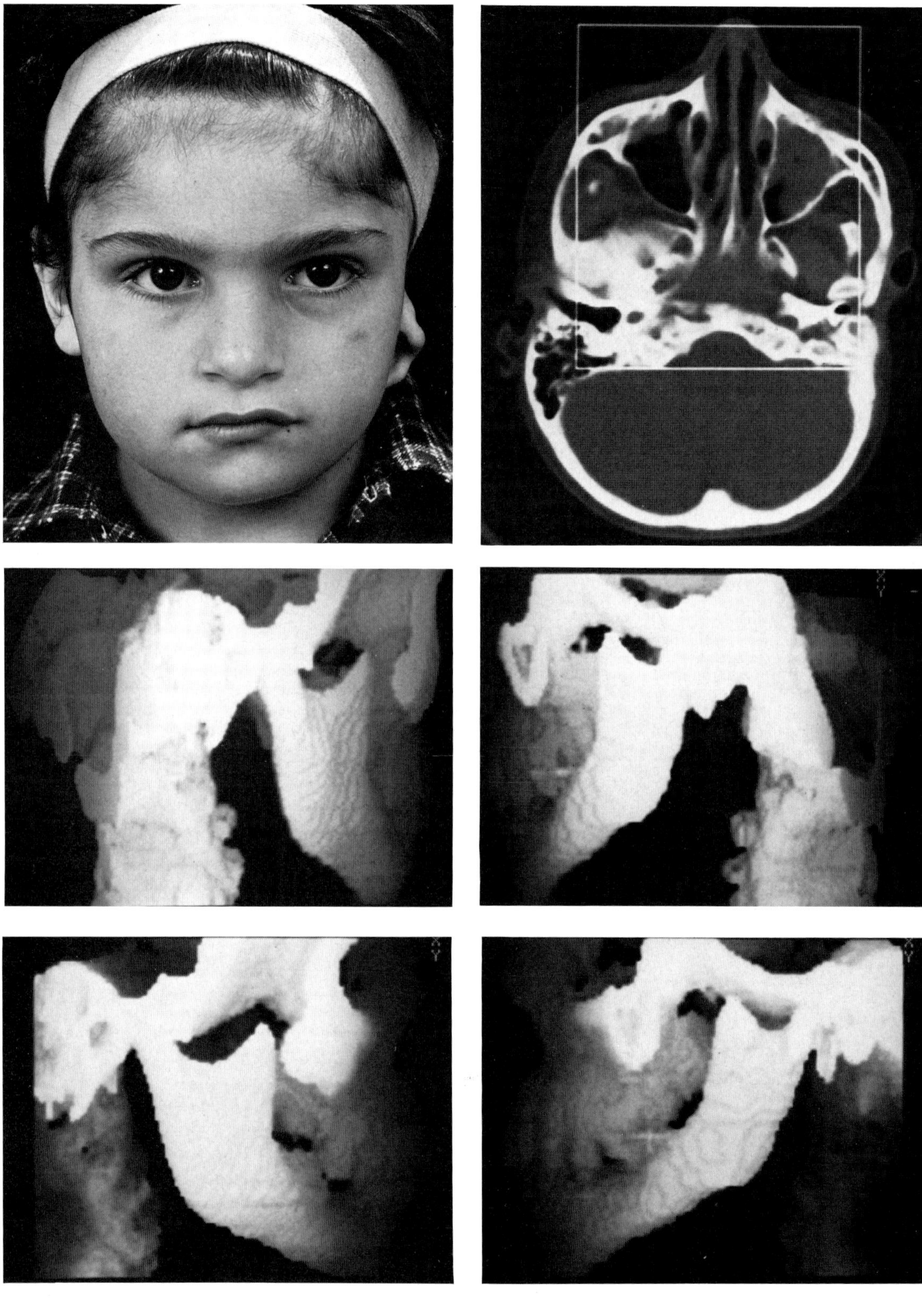

A B C D E F

A B C D

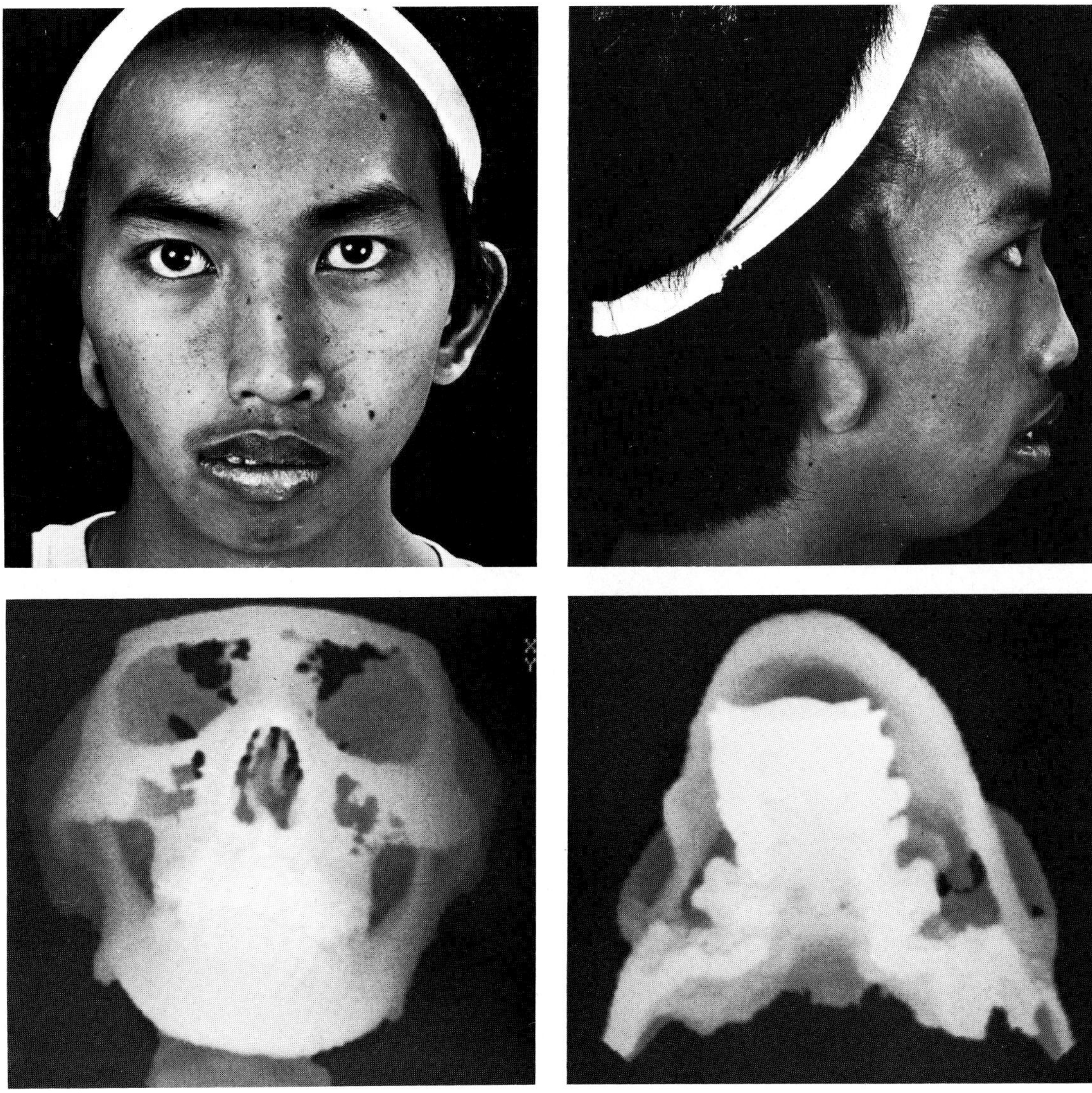

Fig. 5.19. A Craniofacial microsomia patients with minimal skeletal deformity may have a severe microtia. This patient has a deformity classified $S_1A_3T_1$. **B** Using the technique of subregioning, only the bony elements within the box cursor are included in a subsequent three-dimensional reconstruction. **C,D** Comparative views of this patient's mandibular rami (zygomatic arches excluded from the three-dimensional image) show the reduced height of the left mandibular ramus, consistent with a type S_1 skeletal deformity. **E,F** Lateral views of the mandible further highlight the smaller size but relatively normal shape of the left mandibular ramus.

Fig. 5.20. A,B Distorted ear remnant is the dominant external deformity in this craniofacial microsomia patient with the classification $S_2A_3T_2$. **C** Shortening of the right mandibular ramus with some distortion of the temporomandibular joint make it a type S_2 mandible. **D** Viewed from below, the mandibular asymmetry can be seen clearly. This view is also useful for demonstrating differences in size and shape of the temporomandibular joint.

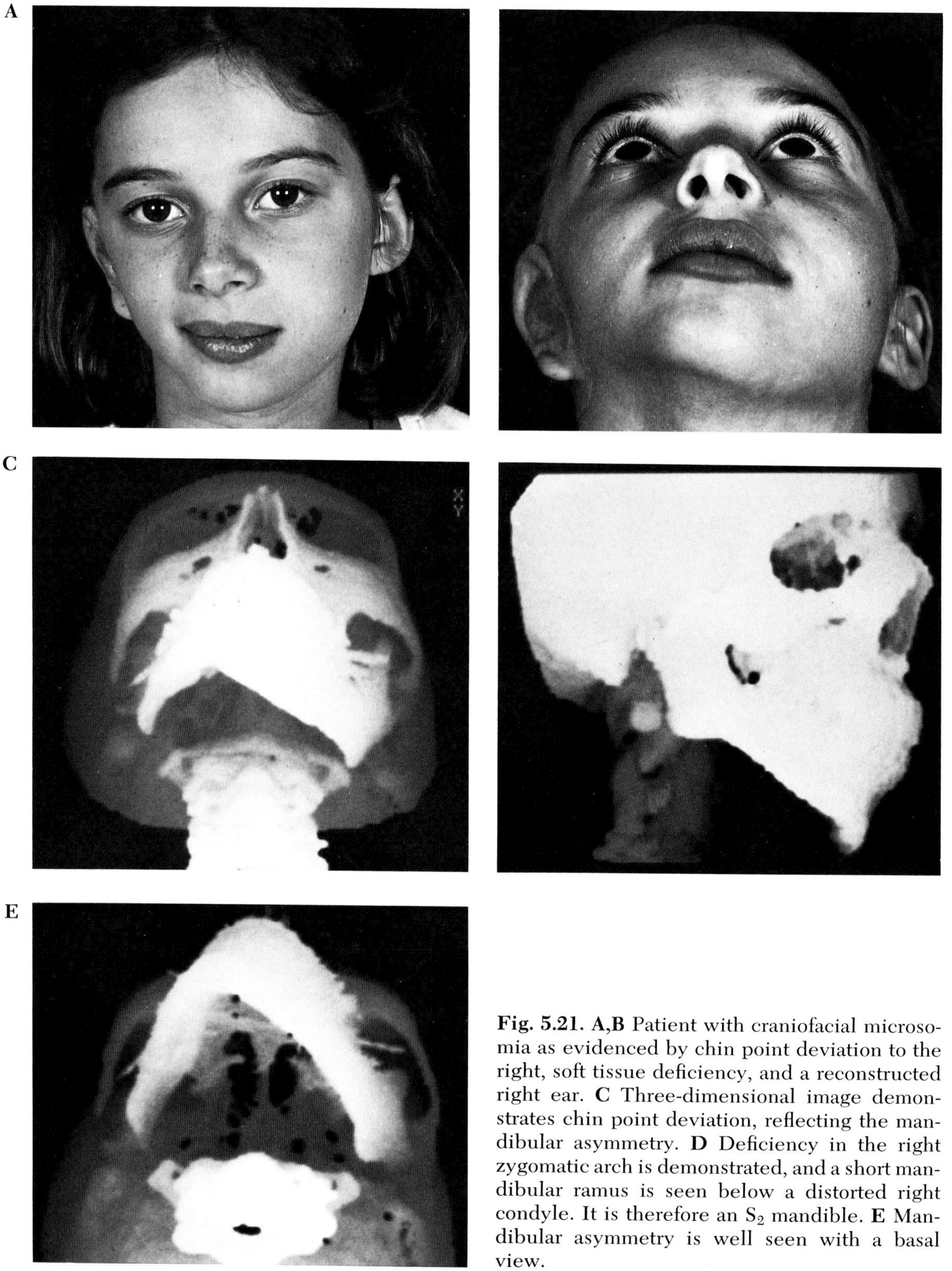

Fig. 5.21. **A,B** Patient with craniofacial microsomia as evidenced by chin point deviation to the right, soft tissue deficiency, and a reconstructed right ear. **C** Three-dimensional image demonstrates chin point deviation, reflecting the mandibular asymmetry. **D** Deficiency in the right zygomatic arch is demonstrated, and a short mandibular ramus is seen below a distorted right condyle. It is therefore an S_2 mandible. **E** Mandibular asymmetry is well seen with a basal view.

A

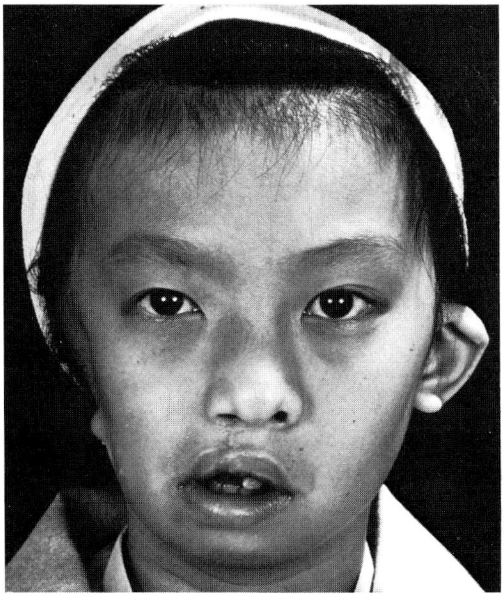

B

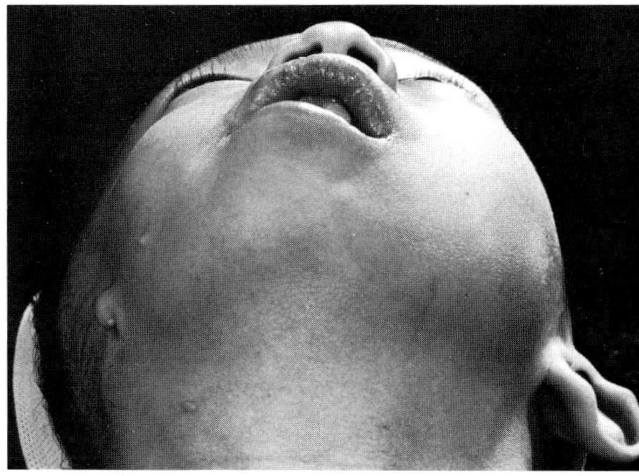

D

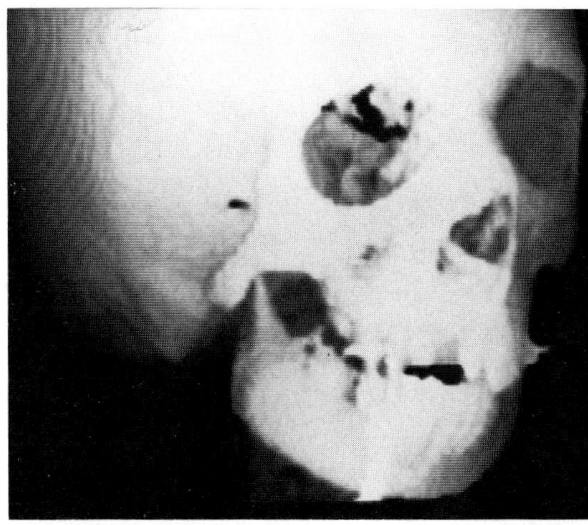

C

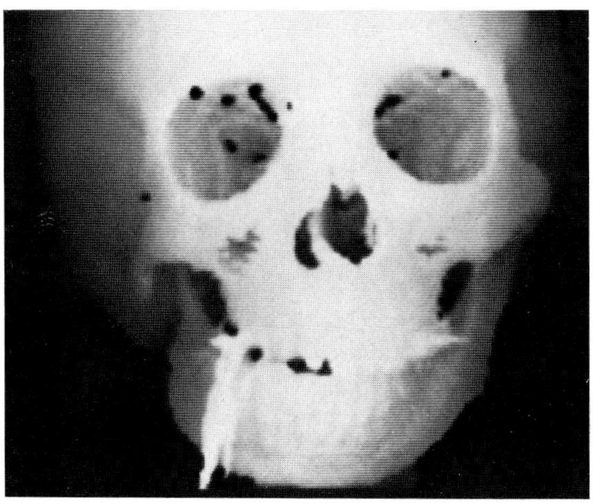

E

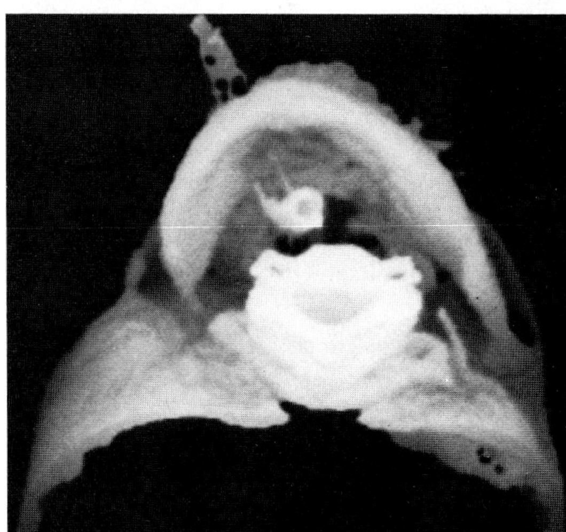

Fig. 5.22. **A** Anotia on the right with significant soft tissue deficiency, chin point deviation to the right, and a repaired right cleft lip and palate make this craniofacial microsomia $S_3A_3T_3$. (Refer also to Figure 5.8.) **B** Viewed from below, the degree of asymmetry is well seen. **C** Right mandibular ramus consists of a thin bony spur consistent with a type S_3 skeletal deformity. **D** Right zygomatic arch is deficient. **E** Viewed from below, the mandibular midline is deviated to the right, and the right condyle and ramus are absent.

A B C D

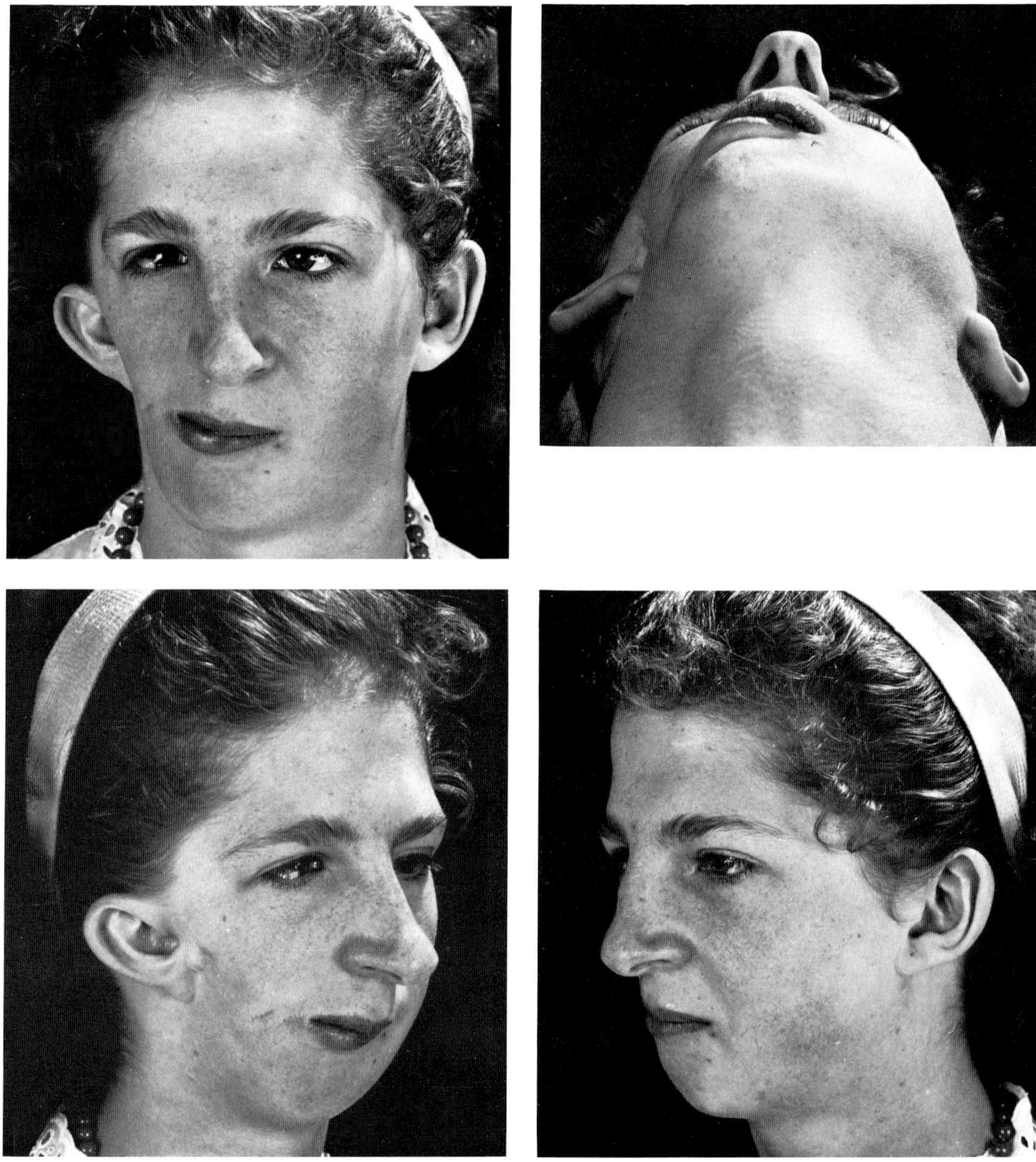

Fig. 5.23. A Severe Goldenhar syndrome with an epibulbar cyst and right craniofacial microsomia ($S_4A_1T_3$). **B** Gross deviation of the chin and loss of soft tissue on the right side with malposition of the right ear. **C,D** Oblique photographs show the difference between the two sides of the face. **E** Soft tissue structures can be reconstructed with the three-dimensional reconstruction program. **F** Standard orthopantomogram revealed the absence of the right mandibular ramus. **G** Note the gross deficiency of the right side of the mandible, absence of the temporomandibular joint, absence of the zygomatic arch, and hypoplasia of the maxilla. There is orbital and skull base asymmetry. **H** Oblique view demonstrates distortion of the lateral orbital wall together with the lack of bony development on the right side from the base of the skull to the mandibular body. It is a skeletal type S_4 deformity with posterior recession of the lateral orbital wall. **I** Viewed from below, the absence of right mandibular elements is clearly seen.

E

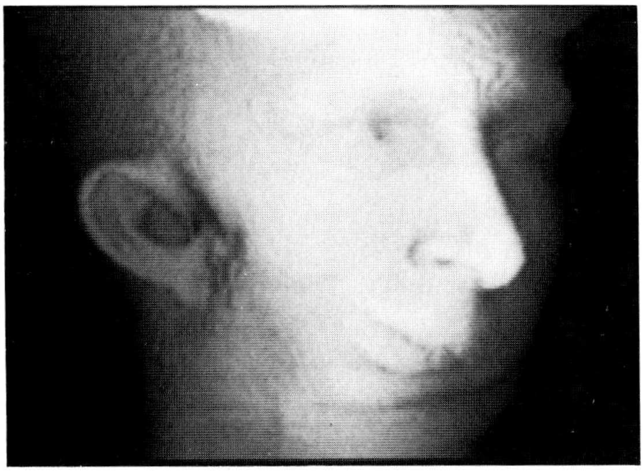

F

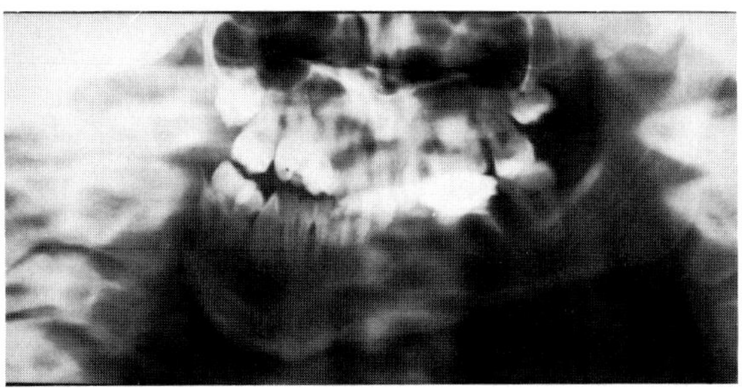

G

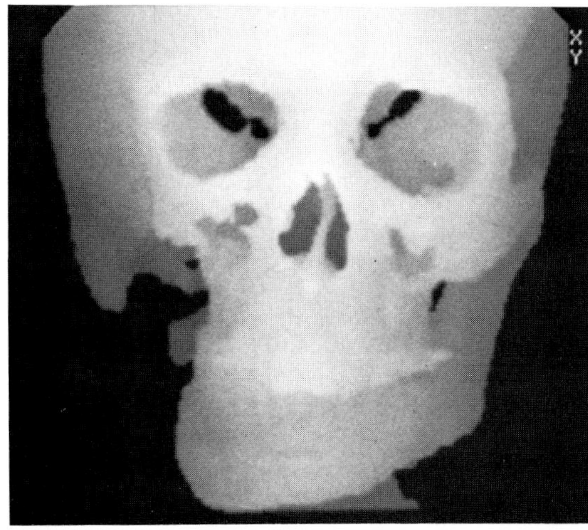

H

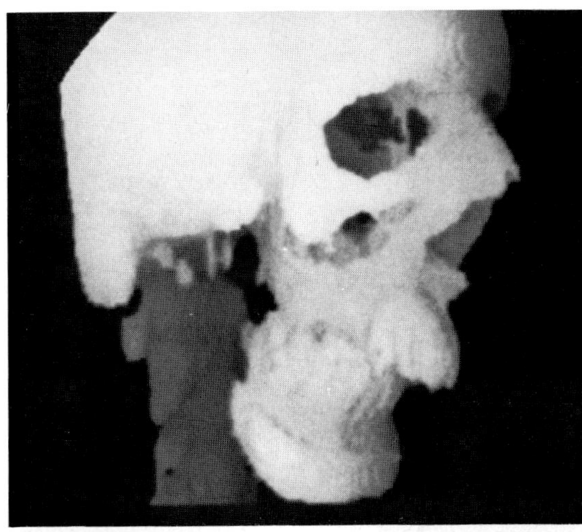

I

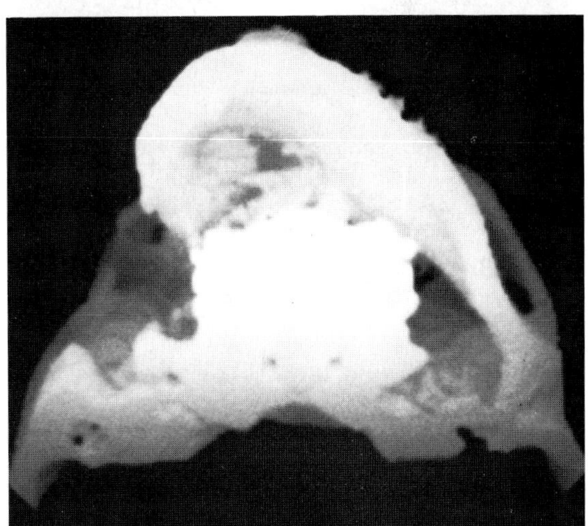

A

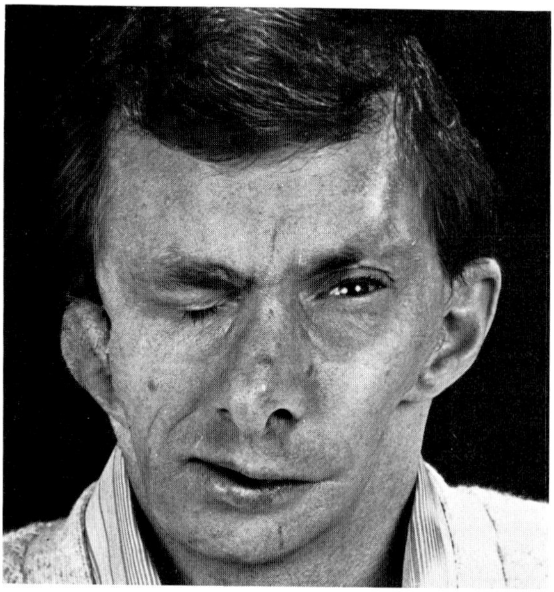

B

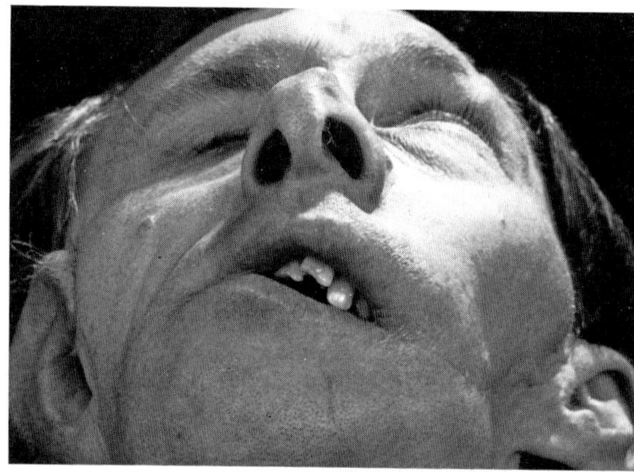

C

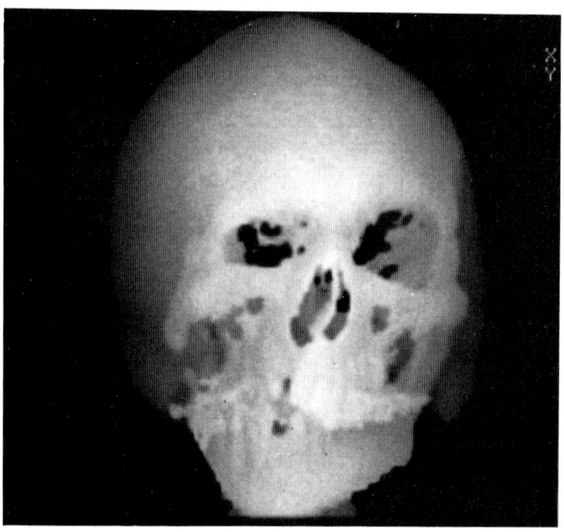

D

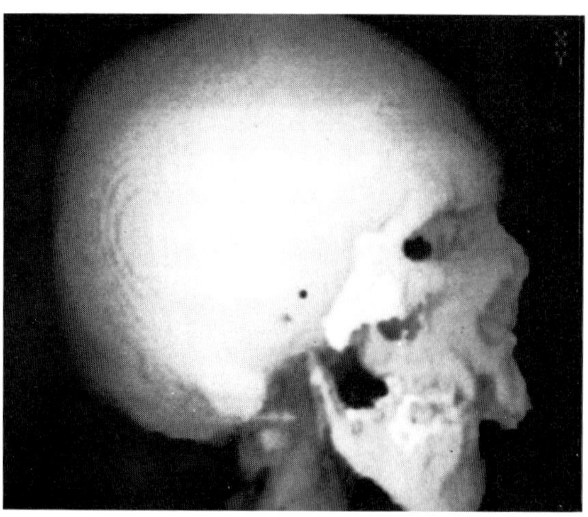

E

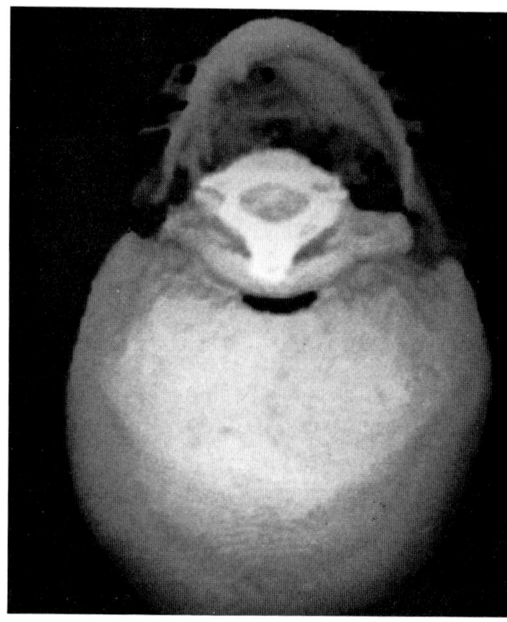

Fig. 5.24. A,B Severe form of craniofacial microsomia may be associated with orbital hypoplasia and severe soft tissue deficiency. This patient also has a poorly sited right ear reconstruction and a soft tissue cleft extending from the left eyebrow up to the hairline. **C** Orbital hypoplasia in association with a severe mandibular deformity make this patient's skeletal classification type S_5. **D** Right lateral three-dimensional image shows a small orbit, absence of the zygomatic arch, absence of the temporomandibular joint, and absence of both the condyle and coronoid process of the mandible. The small bony extension in the position of the right condyle is a remnant of a bone graft from a previous attempt at reconstruction. **E** There is a lack of development of the base of the skull on the affected side together with absence of the zygomatic arch and temporomandibular joint.

6

Meningoencephaloceles

A congenital meningoencephalocele is a herniation of brain and meninges through a skull defect. Meningoencephaloceles may be categorized as occipital, parietal, basal, and sincipital lesions. The latter group has been further classified by Suwanwela and Suwanwela (1972), based on a paper by von Meyer (1890), as: (1) frontoethmoidal (nasofrontal, nasoethmoidal, and nasoorbital), (2) interfrontal, and (3) craniofacial clefts.

Frontoethmoidal Meningoencephalocele

The term "frontoethmoidal" is appropriate because it describes the site of the cranial end of the defect, which is always through the foramen cecum at the junction of the frontal (membranous) and ethmoidal (cartilaginous) bones (Figs. 6.1–6.4). It is through this bony defect in the region of the foramen cecum that a herniation of brain tissue extends to the root of the nose (Fig. 6.1A,B) or the orbit (Fig. 6.4A). The posterior margin of the defect is formed by the crista galli (Figs. 6.1F and 6.2D). It is often distorted, and the cribriform plate is usually tilted downward (Fig. 6.1D) as a deep central trough, the anterior end of which is well below the planum sphenoidale. The cribriform plate forms an angle of 45°–50° with the orbitomeatal plane. In all cases the face appears to be longer than normal, and the piriform aperture and nasal cartilages are misshapen. Some patients have dental malocclusion, which may be related to the deformity: The vertical plate of the ethmoid bone is attached to the tilted cribriform plate, which is itself retrodisplaced (Fig. 6.1F), presumably inducing secondary maxillary hypoplasia. The pathological constituents of the herniations vary. Some patients have viable brain at the neck of the encephalocele, but distal to the defect in the dura mater biopsies generally show glial tissue. The soft tissue mass of the meningoencephalocele may extend into the orbits and fuse with the periorbitum. The facial component of the defect determines the subclassifications: nasofrontal, nasoethmoidal, and nasoorbital.

Nasofrontal Defect

With a nasofrontal deformity, the skull defect presents at the root of the nose, pushing the nasal bones inferiorly (Fig. 6.1C,D). There are varying degrees of lateral displacement of the medial orbital walls. The cribriform plate and crista galli are tilted downward (Fig. 6.1D), producing a deep anterior fossa centrally (Fig. 6.1F).

Nasoethmoidal Defect

With the nasoethmoidal deformity, the anterior cranial fossa defect is similar to the nasofrontal variety, but the facial defect lies between the nasal bones and the nasal cartilages below (Fig. 6.2B,C). The nasal bones are deformed and often broadened with crimped margins. If the facial defect is confined to the nasal pyramid and is small and oval, the medial walls of the orbit are not involved. If the meningoencephalocele is larger and the facial defect extends more laterally, however, the anterior margins of the medial orbital walls are eroded and become crescent-shaped.

Nasoorbital Defect

The nasoorbital deformity reaches the face through holes in the medial orbital walls situated in the frontal process of the maxilla and the lacrimal bones (Figs. 6.3C,D and 6.4B,C). The bony tract is long and shaped like an inverted Y, and the defect may be asymmetrical. The meningoencephalocele protrudes through the frontal process of the maxilla onto the face (Figs. 6.3A,B and 6.4A), leaving the nasal bone intact anteriorly (Fig. 6.3E) and the lacrimal bone and lateral plate of the ethmoid intact posteriorly (Fig. 6.4B,C). During its passage through the substance of the ethmoid, the lateral plate is pushed laterally, with a bony tunnel being formed by these cranial contents (Fig. 6.4D).

Basal Meningoencephalocele

The basal meningoencephalocele (Figs. 6.5 and 6.6) herniates through a defect in the skull base (Figs. 6.5B,C and 6.6C,D). This deformity may be subclassified as follows.

Intranasal—in which the hernia passes through the cribriform plate into the nasal cavity (Figs. 6.5 and 6.6).

Sphenopharyngeal—passing through the sphenoid bone and presenting as a mass in the pharynx.

Sphenoorbital—traversing the superior orbital fissure to enter the orbit.

Sphenomaxillary—an extended sphenoorbital type with the mass continuing through the inferior orbital fissure into the pterygopalatine fossa and presenting as a mass on the medial side of the ramus of the mandible.

Recommended Reading

David DJ, Sheffield L, Simpson D, White J: Fronto-ethmoidal meningoencephaloceles: morphology and treatment. Br J Plast Surg 37:271, 1984.

Hang Thur, Hta Kyu: Epidemiology of fronto-ethmoidal encephalomeningocele in Burma. J Epidemiol Commun Health 38:89, 1984.

Hemmy DC, David DJ: Skeletal morphology of anterior encephalocele defined through the use of three-dimensional reconstruction of computed tomography. Paediatr Neurosci 12:18, 1985–1986.

Hemmy DC, David DJ, Herman GT: Three-dimensional reconstruction of craniofacial deformity using computed tomography. Neurosurgery 13:534, 1983.

Naim-Ur-Rahman: Naso-encephalocele: treatment by transcranial operation. J Neurol Sci 42:73, 1979.

Simpson DA, David DJ, White J: Cephaloceles: treatment, outcome and antenatal diagnosis. Neurosurgery 15:14, 1984.

Suwanwela C: Geographic distribution of fronto-ethmoidal encephalomeningocele. Br J Prev Soc Med 26:193, 1972.

Suwanwela C, Sukabote C, Suwanwela N: Fronto-ethmoidal encephalomeningocele. Surgery 69:617, 1971.

Suwanwela C, Suwanwela N: A morphological classification of sincipital encephaloceles. J Neurosurg 36:201, 1972.

Tessier P: Orbital hypertelorism: successive surgical attempts, materials and methods, causes and mechanisms. Scand J Plast Reconstr Surg 6:135, 1972.

Von Meyer E: Über eine basale Hirnhernie in der Gegend der Lamina Cribosa. Virchows Arch [Pathol Anat] 120:309, 1890.

Fig. 6.1. A,B Large frontoethmoidal meningoencephalocele with protrusion of dysplastic brain covered by pigmented skin. The mass distorts the upper and middle face. **C** There is widening of the interorbital distance but relative normality of the lateral orbital walls. The distortion produced by the mass is reflected in the altered orbital shapes. This deformity is the nasofrontal variety because the nasal bones are below the exit hole on the face. The cribriform plate and crista galli can be seen in the depths of the defect. **D** Oblique view demonstrates the exit hole

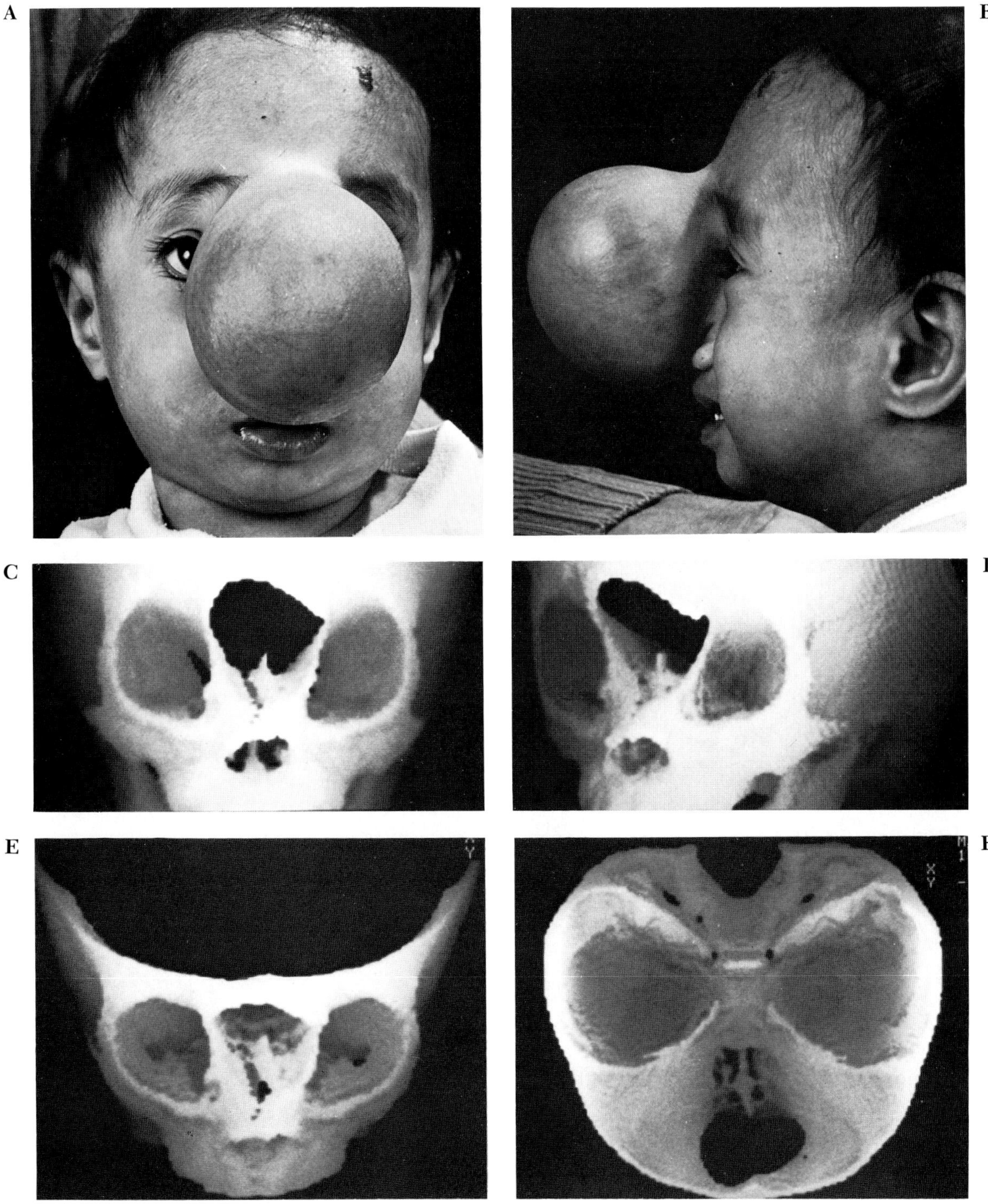

and its relation with the base of the skull. The cribriform plate is depressed; its relations with the right medial orbital wall and right orbital roof are well demonstrated. **E** Piriform aperture is displaced caudally and distorted by the emerging mass of brain tissue. **F** View into the anterior cranial fossa shows the exit hole at the site of the foramen cecum, anterior to the crista galli. The anterior fossa is depressed centrally, and the cribriform plate is widened.

A B C D

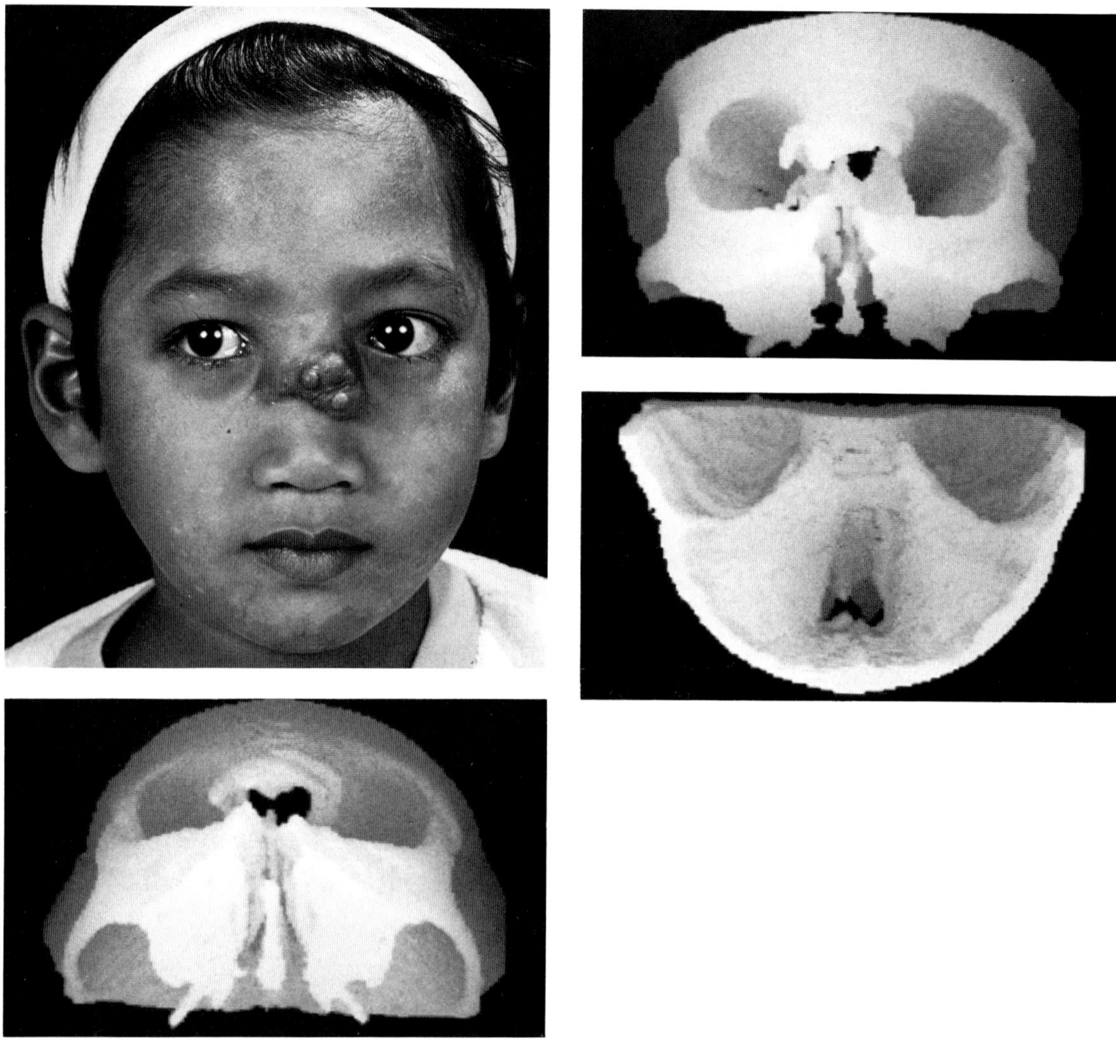

Fig. 6.2. A With the nasoethmoidal type of frontoethmoidal meningoencephalocele there is no general hypertelorism, but the patient has a long face and mild telecanthus. The skin over the nasal bridge is altered. **B,C** The side of the departure is situated below the nasal bones, which are shortened and distorted with crenated margins. There is no genuine hypertelorism in this instance. There is a false accentuation of the frontozygomatic suture due to lateral movement of the patient during the scan. **D** Bilobed exit hole from the anterior cranial fossa is a common finding with this type of meningoencephalocele. It is usually sited anterior to the crista galli, at the foramen cecum.

Fig. 6.3. A,B This patient has a nasoorbital frontoethmoidal meningoencephalocele with an elongated face and a mass protruding onto the right side of the nose and extending into the lower part of the right orbit. **C,D** Osseous image shows an intact piriform margin deviated to the left. There is widening of the intercanthal region and distortion of the medial orbital wall, but the lateral orbital walls are in normal position. The encephalocele distorts the medial orbital wall in the region of the lacrimal bone and the frontal process of the maxilla. **E** Oblique view demonstrates the defect in the right medial orbital wall. **F** Anterior cranial fossa view shows the bilobed exit hole. ▶

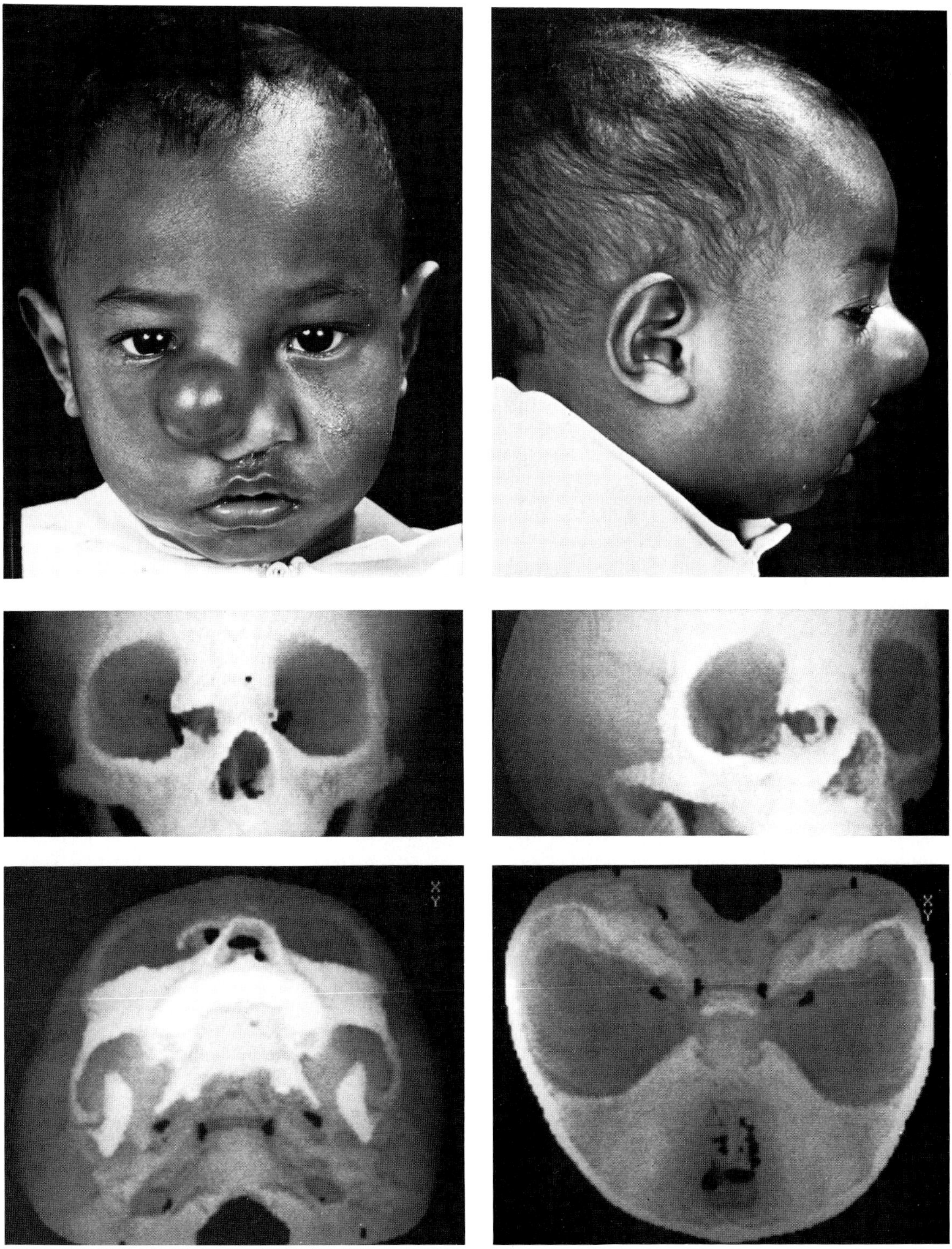

A B C E D F

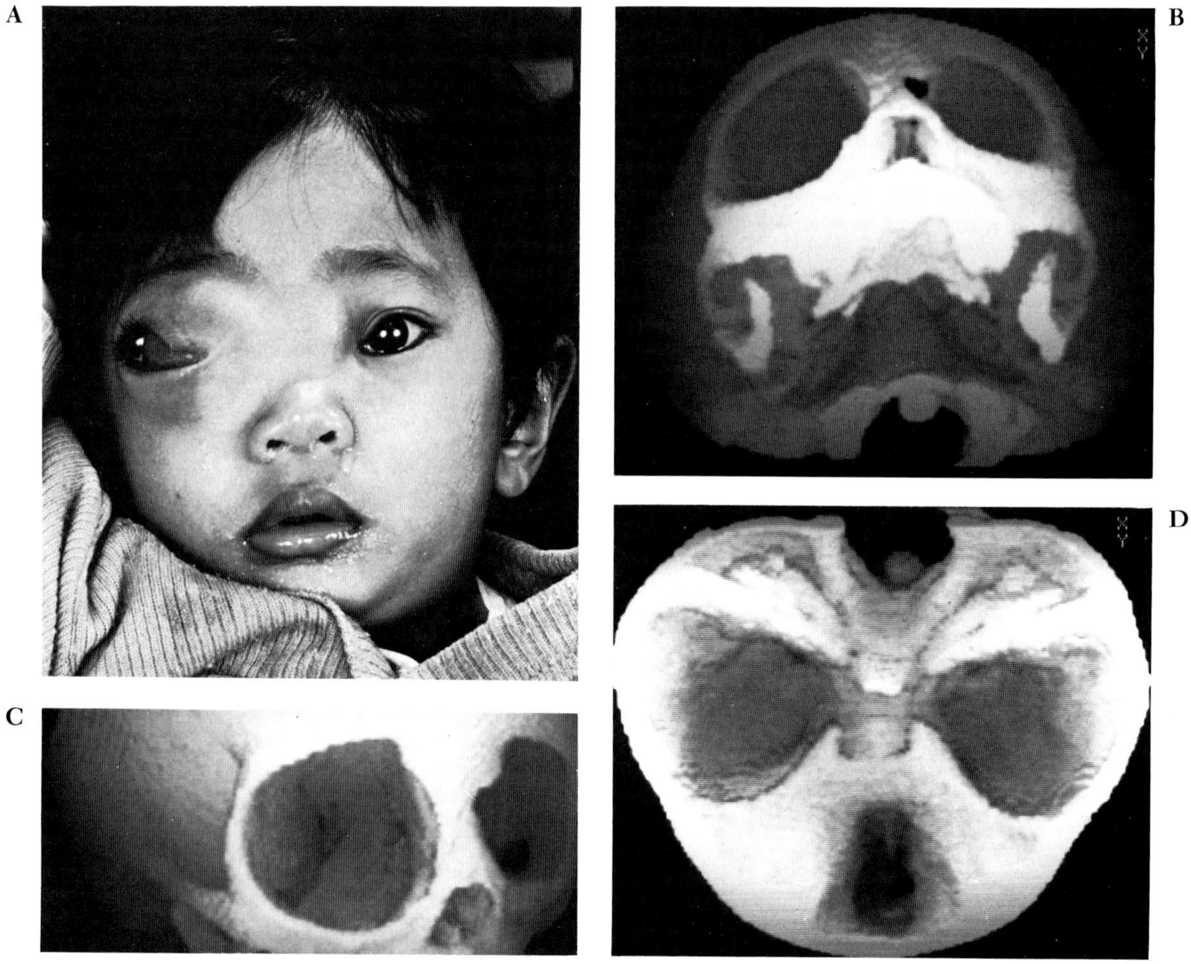

Fig. 6.4. A Nasoorbital variety of frontoethmoidal meningoencephalocele in which the bulk of the extruded cerebral tissue has herniated into the right orbit, expanding the orbit and displacing the globe. There is little longitudinal distortion of this patient's face. **B,C** Small foramen is seen to the left of the midline through which a small amount of brain emerges. The greatest penetration of brain is seen in the right orbit, however, expanding it. **D** The cribriform plate is markedly depressed, with a wide exit foramen anteriorly. One can see a small departure site on the left and a longer tunnel on the right. This case provides a good example of how the displaced brain deforms the developing bones of the face, which are not primarily dysplastic.

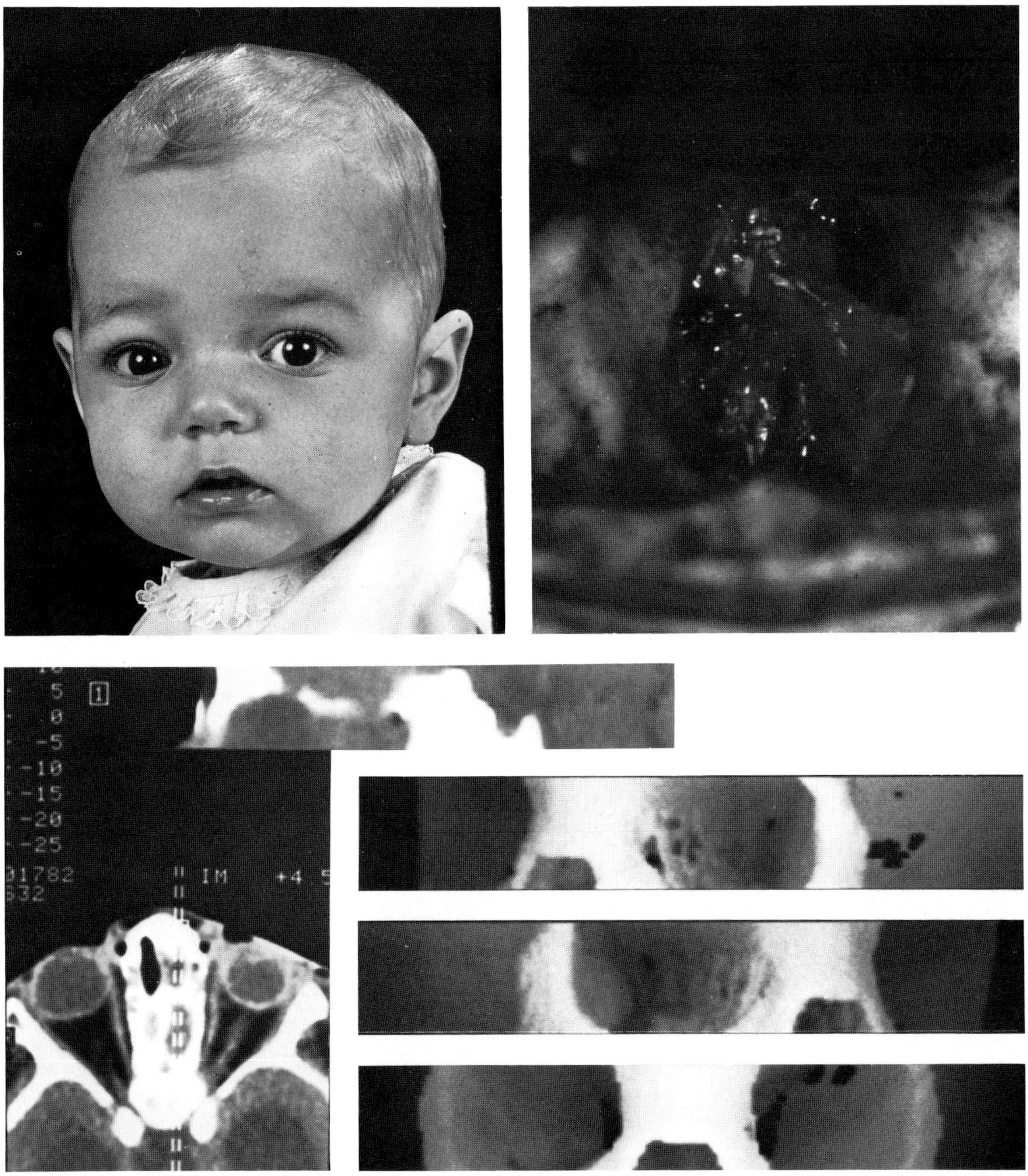

Fig. 6.5. **A** Patients with basal encephaloceles usually have a normal facial appearance. **B** Operative photograph looking into the anterior cranial fossa clearly shows the basal encephalocele's exit hole through the posterior aspect of the cribriform plate on the patient's left. **C** Sagittal section through the cribriform plate further demonstrates the exit hole behind the crista galli. **D–F** Series of limited three-dimensional images demonstrating the symmetrically intact orbital walls.

A B

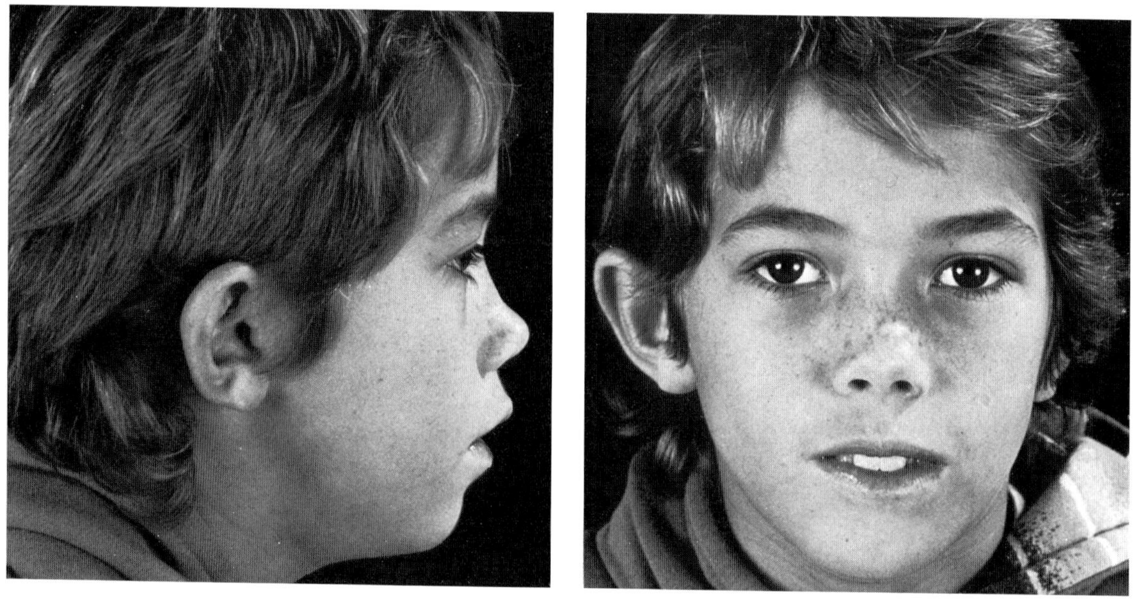

C

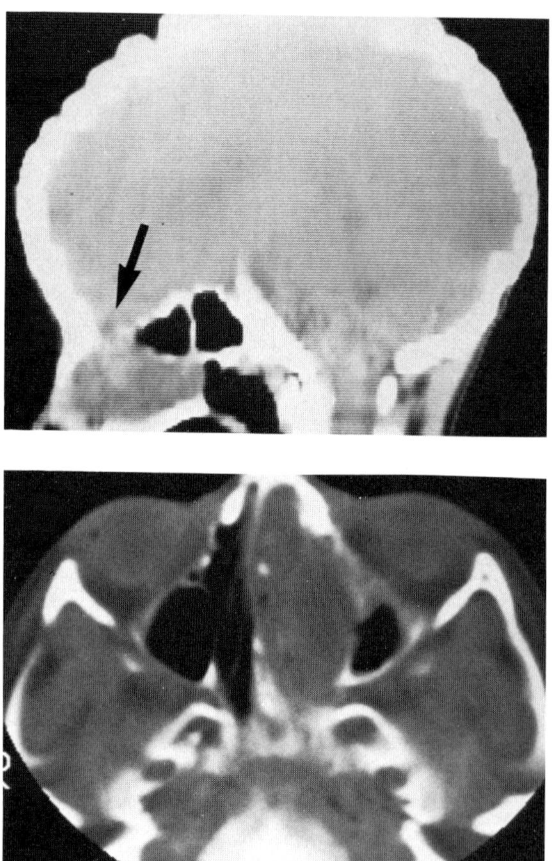

D

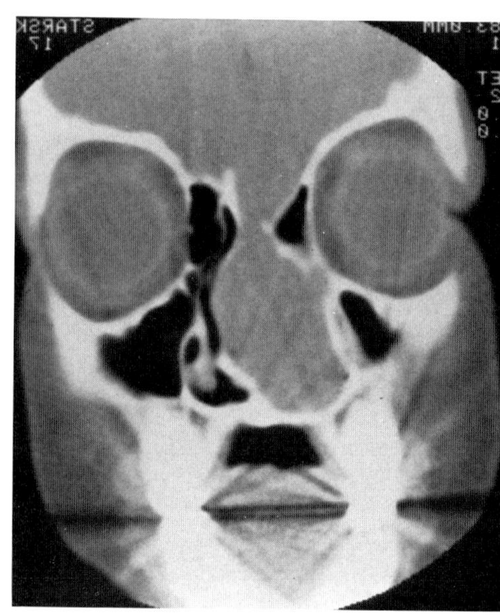

E

Fig. 6.6. A,B Basal encephalocele has filled the posterior nasal space on the left, but there is no overt deformity. **C** Encephalocele has herniated through the floor of the anterior fossa to enter the nasal cavity. **D** Coronal reformat shows the brain herniation lateral to the crista galli. **E** Axial slice at the level of the zygomatic arches. The left nasal cavity has been filled with the basal encephalocele.

7

Growth Disorders

Growth disorders such as microorbitism, Binder syndrome, Romberg syndrome, and radiation effects are often difficult to quantify because they have unpredictable rates of distortion with time. The three-dimensional appreciation of the deformity needs to be imaged sequentially over a period of time. It is important to consider volume measurements, particularly of the orbits, for these disease entities, as well as shape analyses with comparisons made between normal and abnormal sides.

Primary Growth Disorders

Microorbitism

A small orbit is a general response to hypoplasia or aplasia of the orbital contents. It may be congenital or acquired. It can occur as an isolated event (Fig. 7.1) or in association with other craniofacial abnormalities, particularly the clefts (Figs. 7.2 and 7.3).

The currently accepted thesis is that the eye, like the brain, grows rapidly during the first 2 years of life. Its bony covering, the orbit, responds similarly to the way in which the calvaria responds to rapid brain growth. Absence of this drive produces a small orbit.

In most instances, the presence of a microphthalmic eye of varying degrees of development may be accompanied by an orbital deformity that may not be marked. However, in the true anophthalmic orbit the deformity is a failure of orbital growth with a small bony orbit that manifests as a depression of the anterior cranial fossa on the affected side and a degree of hypertelorism involving the medial orbital wall. Maxillary hypoplasia of that side is also common.

Binder Syndrome

The syndrome "dysostosis maxillonasalis" was first described by Binder in 1962. The condition is characterized by a flat midface with concomitant flattening of the nose and obliteration of the nasofrontal angle (Fig. 7.4). There is hypoplasia of the anterior nasal spine (Fig. 7.4C,D), and the frontal sinuses are often hypoplastic. As a result of maxillary retrusion, there is pseudomandibular prognathism with class III malocclusion (Figs. 7.4B–D), although in some cases the occlusion is normal. Some cases that demonstrate a hereditary tendency have been identified, although it is not usual. The syndrome appears to be part of the wider pattern of chondrodysplasia punctata.

Secondary Growth Disorders

Romberg Syndrome

The Romberg syndrome was described by Parry and Romberg during the first half of the nineteenth century. There is progressive atrophy of the soft tissues on one side of the face and, rarely, associated atrophy of one-half of the body. The first observed changes often occur in the hair, with poliosis and alopecia affecting eyelashes, eyebrows, and scalp hair. The skin overlying the area of atrophy is pigmented and inelastic (Fig. 7.5A–C). The facial deformity often commences near the midline, and the wasting may involve underlying bone (Fig. 7.5D) as well as subcutaneous fat atrophy (Fig. 7.5A–C). Loss of periorbital fat produces enophthalmos. Deeper structures may also be involved, with resultant hemiatrophy of the tongue and malocclusion.

Radiation Effects

Radiotherapy for tumors in the craniofacial region during infancy may cause significant growth divergence of the irradiated area (Figs. 7.6–7.8). There are atrophic changes in both soft (Figs. 7.6A,B and 7.7A) and hard tissues (Figs. 7.6C, 7.7B–F, and 7.8A–D). Maximal shape distortion occurs if growth centers are included in the irradiated field. Such cases present two major challenges. The tissue changes make difficult any operative intervention, and these patients are at high risk of carcinomatous change in the irradiated area.

Recommended Reading

Ariyan S, Krizek TJ: Radiation effects: biological and surgical considerations. In Converse J (ed): Reconstructive Plastic Surgery. Saunders, Philadelphia, pp 531–548, 1982.

Binder KJ: Dysostosis maxillo-nasalis, ein arhinencephaler Missbildungskomplex. Dtsch Zahnarztl Z 17:438, 1962.

Delaire J, Tessier P, Tulasne JF, Resche F: Clinical and radiologic aspects of maxillonasal dysostosis. Head Neck Surg 3:105, 1980.

Gorlin RJ, Pindborg J, Cohen M Jr (eds): Maxillonasal dysplasia (Binder syndrome). In: Syndromes of the Head and Neck. 2nd ed., McGraw-Hill, New York, pp 463–464, 1976.

Helpin ML, Krejmas NL, Krolls SO: Complications following radiation therapy to the head. Oral Surg Oral Med Oral Pathol 61:209, 1986.

Henderson D, Jackson IT: Naso-maxillary hypoplasia—the Le Fort II osteotomy. Br J Oral Surg 11:77, 1973.

Holmstrom H: Clinical and pathologic features of maxillonasal dysplasia (Binder's syndrome): significance of the prenasal fossa on etiology. Plast Reconstr Surg 78:559, 1986.

Holmstrom H: Surgical correction of the nose and midface in maxillonasal dysplasia (Binder's syndrome). Plast Reconstr Surg 78:568, 1986.

Kawamoto HK Jr: Elective osteotomies and bone grafting of irradiated midfacial bones. J Craniomaxillofac Surg 15:199, 1987.

Mustarde JC: Congenital Absence of the Eye. Saunders, Philadelphia, 1971.

Mustarde JC: Repair and Reconstruction of the Orbital Region. Livingstone, Edinburgh, 1976.

Olow-Nordenram M, Thilander B: The craniofacial morphology in individuals with maxillonasal dysplasia (Binder's syndrome): a longitudinal cephalometric study of orthodontically untreated children. Eur J Orthod 9:224, 1987.

Olow-Nordenram M, Valentin J: An etiologic study of maxillonasal dysplasia—Binder's syndrome. Scand J Dent Res 96:69, 1988.

Parry CH: Collections from the Unpublished Medical Writings of the Late Caleb Hillier Parry. Underwoods, London, p 478, 1825.

Roberts BO: Progressive hemifacial atrophy: Romberg's disease. In Converse J (ed): Reconstructive Plastic Surgery. Saunders, Philadelphia, pp 2337–2353, 1977.

Romberg MH: Trophoneurosen. Klinische Ergebnisse. Forstner, Berlin, pp 75–81, 1846.

Sheffield LJ, White J, David DJ, Nugent M: Chondrodysplasia punctata (mild type) presenting as Binder syndrome. Pathology 16:106, 1984.

Smith B, Valauri AJ: In Converse J (ed): Reconstructive Plastic Surgery. Saunders, Philadelphia, pp 962–980, 1977.

Wood-Smith D: Reconstruction of the orbital skeleton in anophthalmos. In Tessier P, Callahan A, Mustarde JC, Salyer KE (eds): Symposium on Plastic Surgery in the Orbial Region. Mosby, St. Louis, pp 177–179, 1976.

Fig. 7.2. A An anophthalmic orbit was associated with Tessier No. 6 clefts extending into the lower eyelids bilaterally. (Refer also to Figure 5.7.) **B** Plain skull radiograph shows the small orbit on the left. **C** Three-dimensional reconstruction demonstrates a disparity in orbital sizes, with the left being much smaller. The Tessier No. 6 cleft is most obvious on the left and extends from the lateral part of the inferior or-

A

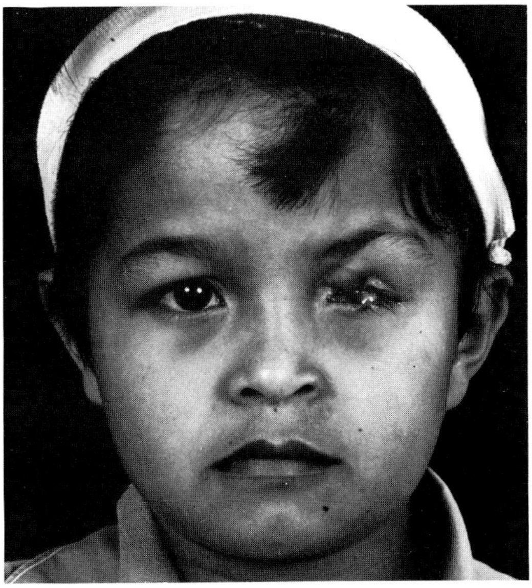

B

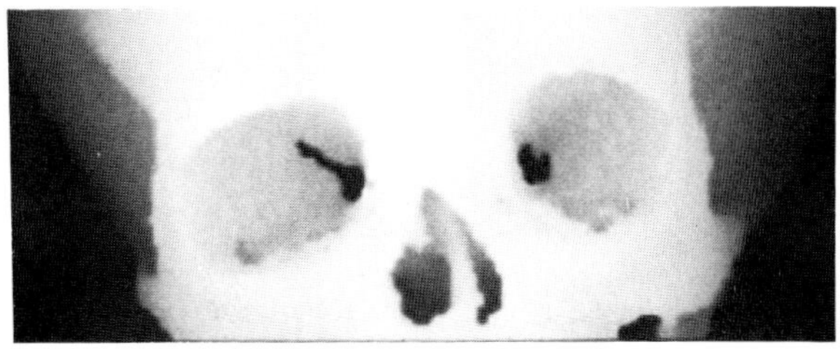

Fig. 7.1. A Anophthalmic orbit may be an isolated finding, as in this otherwise normal Malaysian child. **B** The left orbit is smaller and more globular owing to the lack of a normally expanding globe.

A

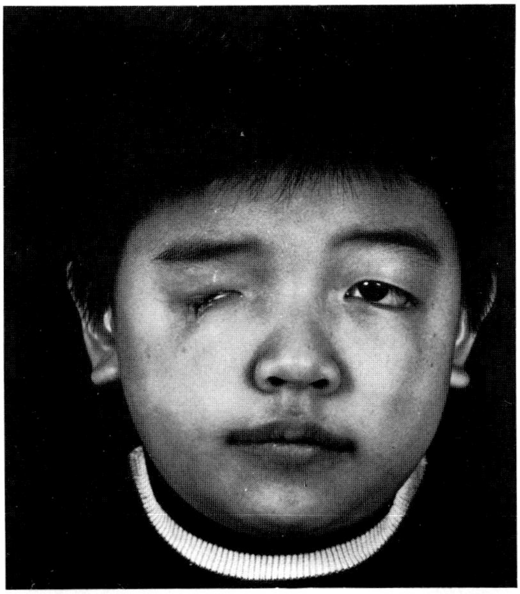

B

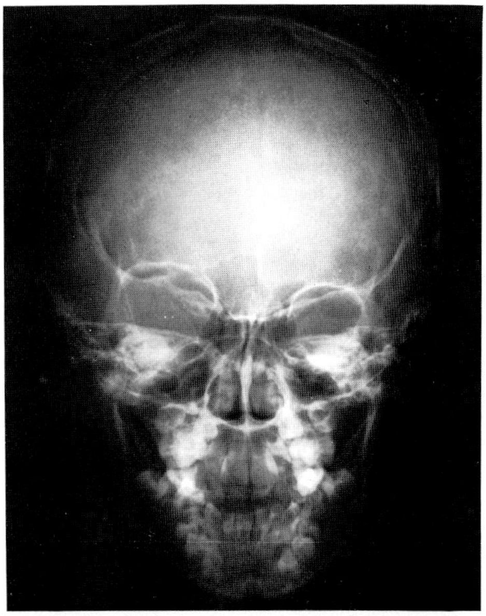

C

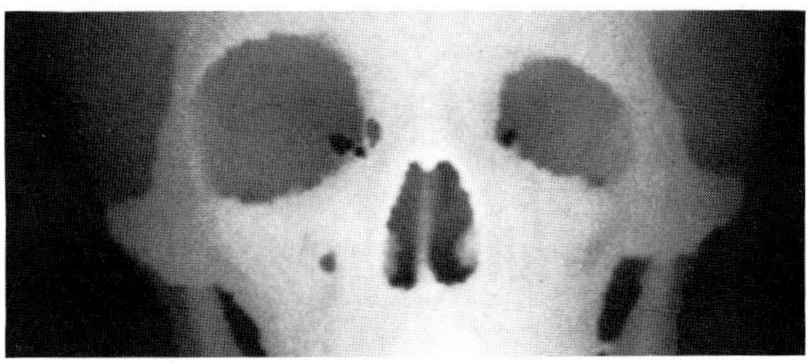

D

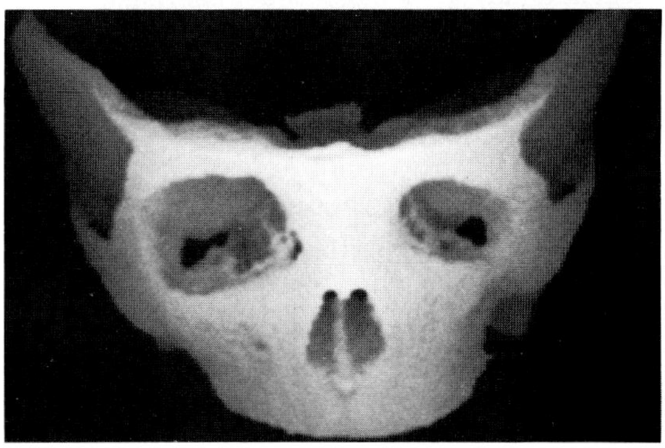

bital margin. **D** Chin-down view demonstrates more clearly the infraorbital margin cleft associated with the microorbitism on the left.

A B C D

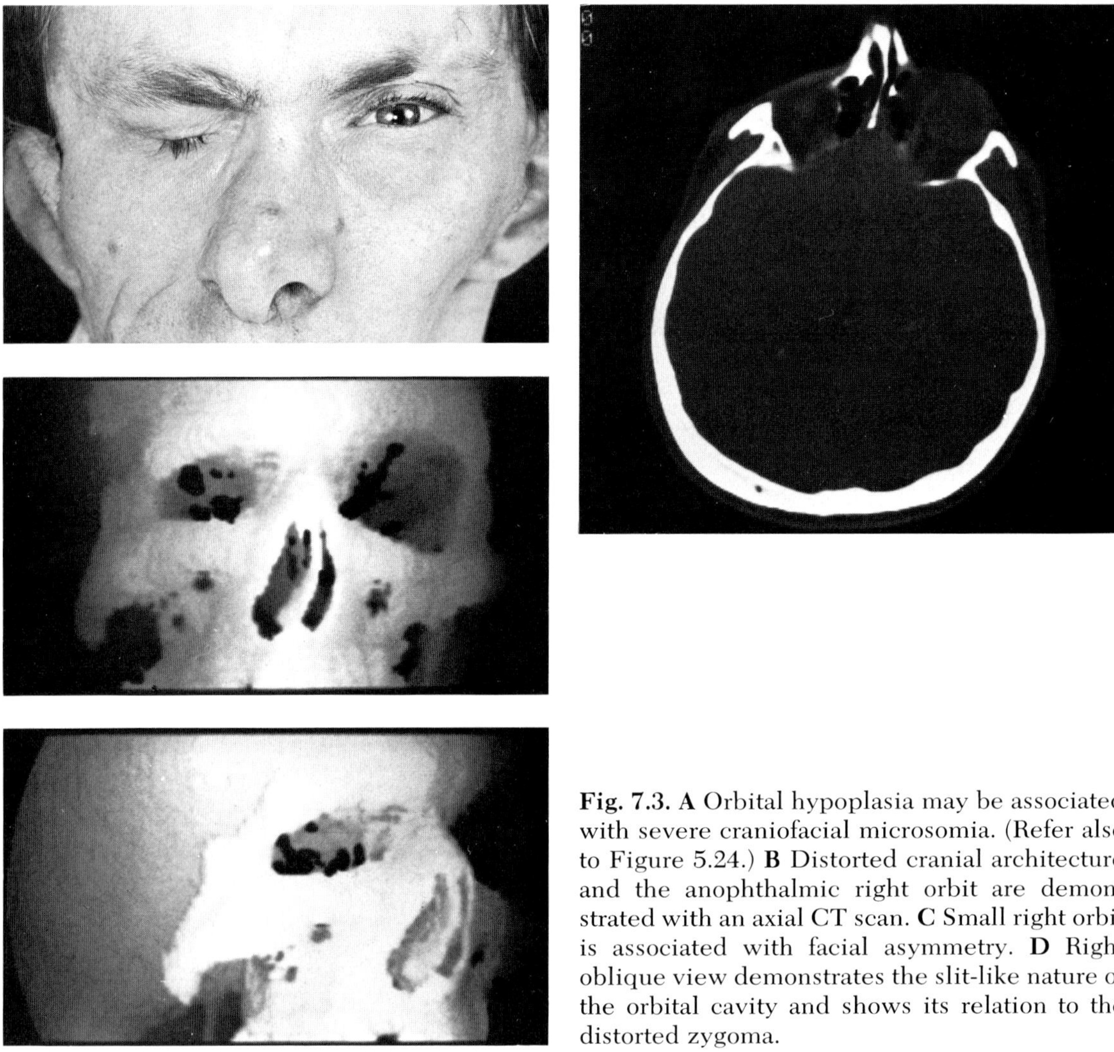

Fig. 7.3. A Orbital hypoplasia may be associated with severe craniofacial microsomia. (Refer also to Figure 5.24.) **B** Distorted cranial architecture and the anophthalmic right orbit are demonstrated with an axial CT scan. **C** Small right orbit is associated with facial asymmetry. **D** Right oblique view demonstrates the slit-like nature of the orbital cavity and shows its relation to the distorted zygoma.

A B

C D

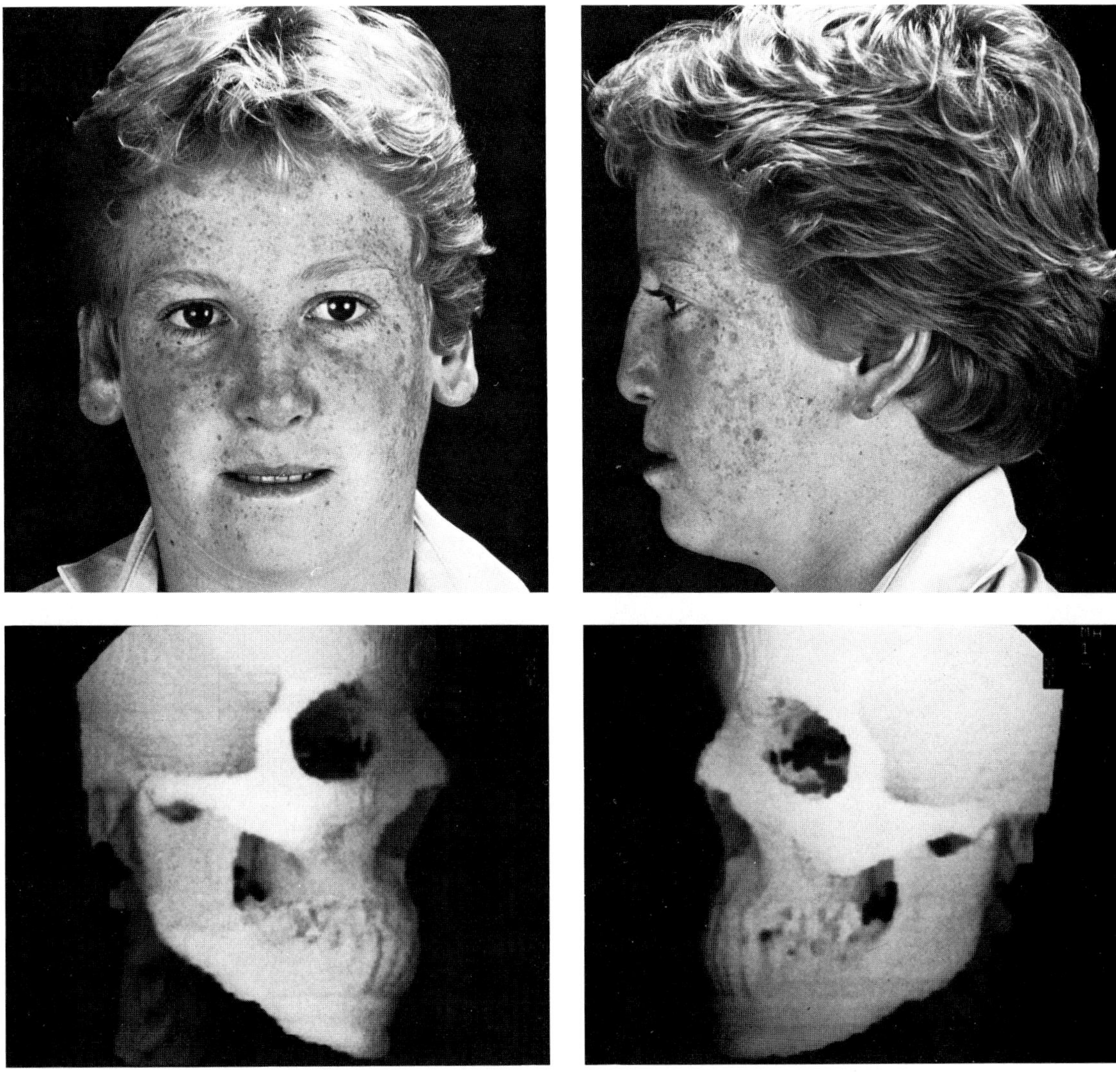

Fig. 7.4. A This boy demonstrates the clinical features of nasomaxillary hypoplasia of Binder. The disorder affects the central part of the midface resulting in a long upper lip that conceals underlying teeth. **B** Lateral view demonstrates the convex upper lip, lack of a nasal spine, typical nasolabial angle, and maxillary hypoplasia with a flat nose. **C,D** On osseous reconstructions the maxilla is seen to be smaller in the region of the hypoplastic nasal spine. There is a class III malocclusion with normal zygomas and a relatively normal nasofrontal angle.

A B

C D

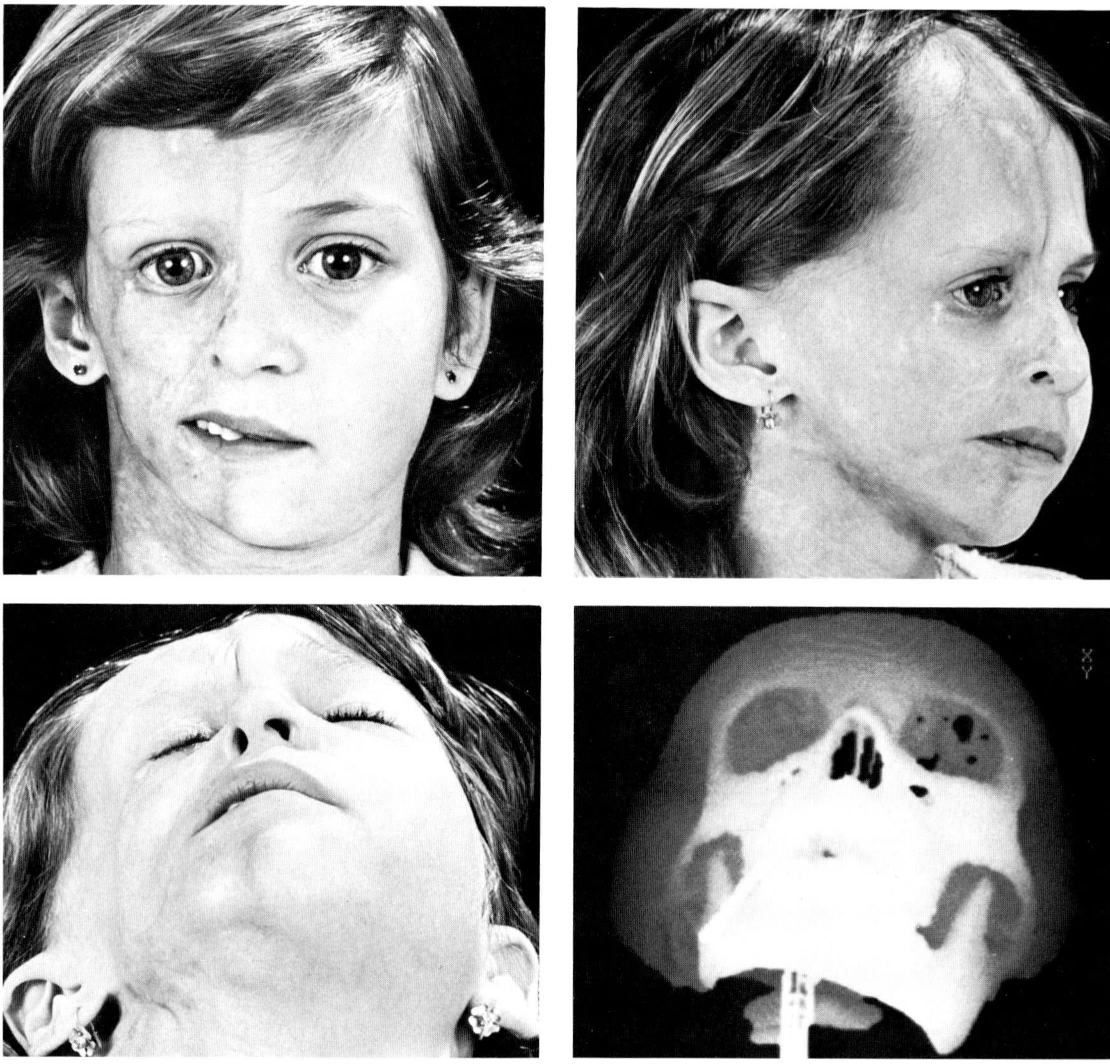

Fig. 7.5. A–C Coup de sabre deformity is clearly seen. The right facial bony contour can be seen through the severely atrophic soft tissues. Poliosis of the right eyebrow and a patch of well demarcated alopecia in the right frontoparietal region are evident. **D** Right-sided atrophy of bony structures affects the upper, middle, and lower facial elements.

A

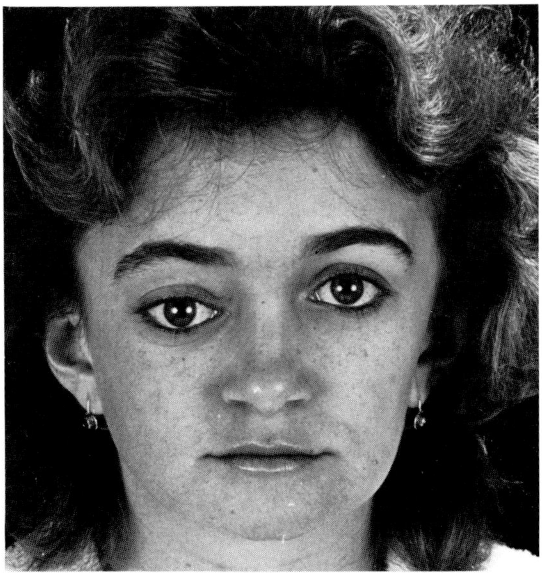

B

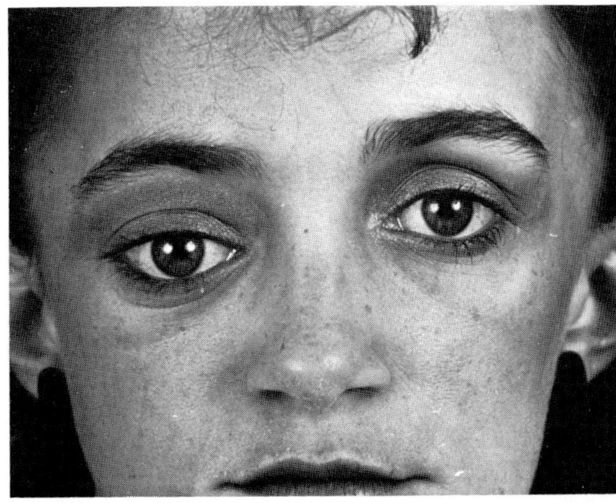

C

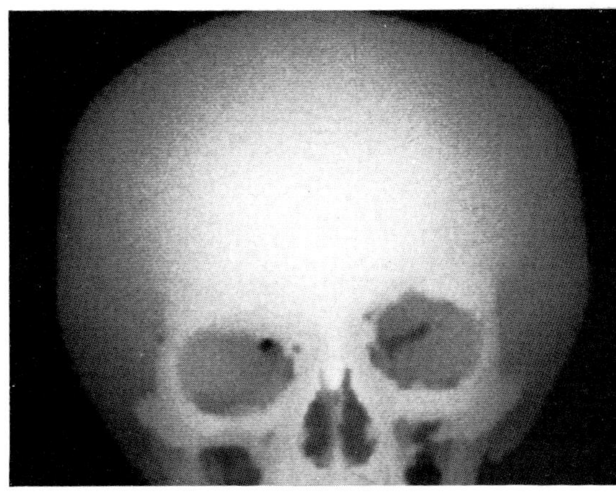

Fig. 7.6. A,B Significant orbital dystopia in this 22-year-old woman followed radiotherapy treatment at 8 years of age for an eosinophilic granuloma. **C** The dystopic right orbit is of normal shape.

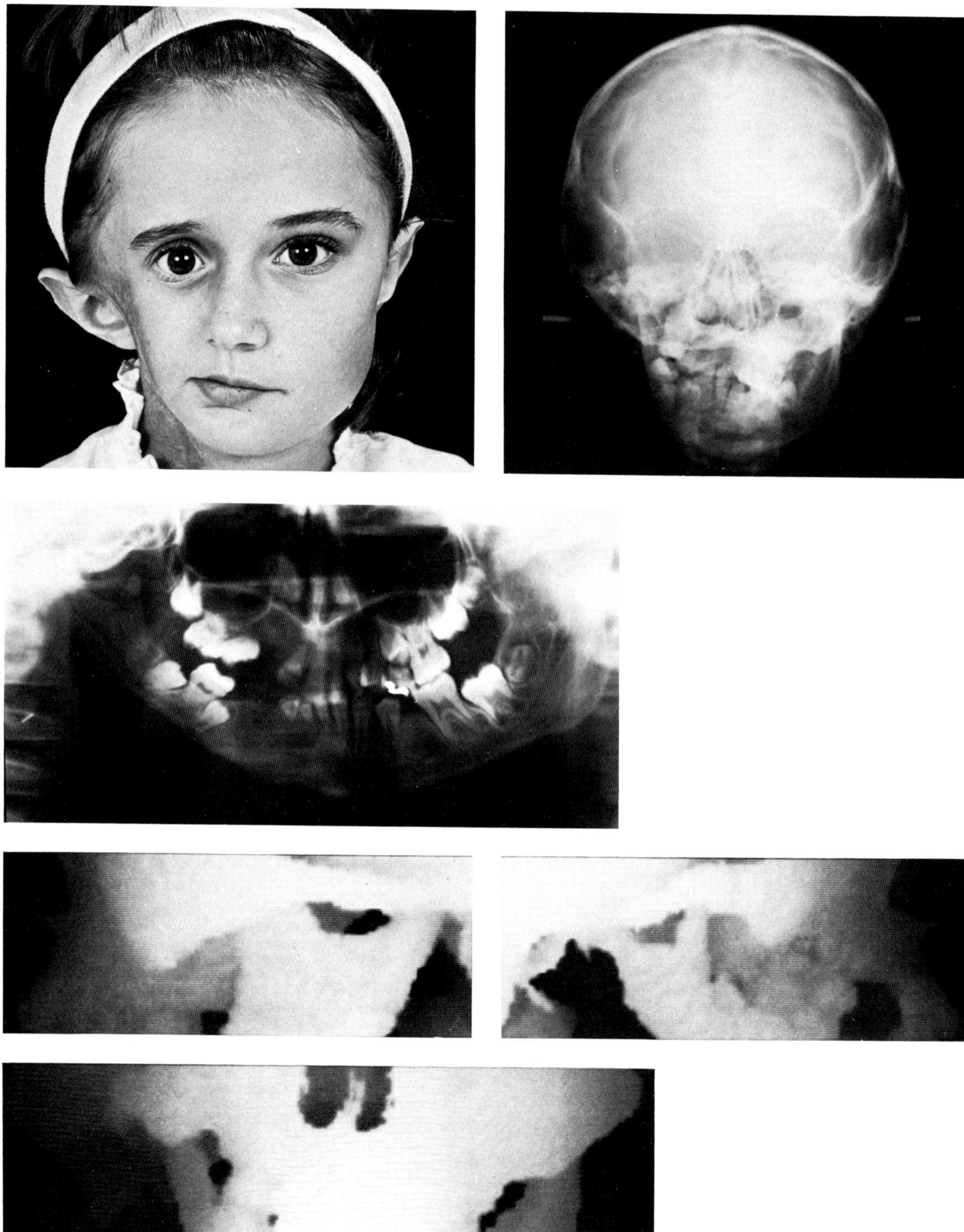

Fig. 7.7. A At 6 weeks of age this 11-year-old girl underwent radiotherapy treatment for a platelet-trapping hemangioma of the face. The secondary hemifacial microsomia is obvious. **B** Facial scoliosis is seen with a plain skull radiograph. **C** Orthopantomogram reveals severe mandibular asymmetry with distortion of the right condyle and coronoid process. **D–F** Comparison of the mandibular rami reveals marked atrophy on the right side due to previous radiotherapy.

Fig. 7.8. A,B Mandibular hypoplasia in a 21-year-old man. At the age of 8 he had had radiotherapy and chemotherapy for a rhabdomyosarcoma of his pharynx. **C,D** The left side is more severely affected. There is chin point deviation to the left and a small ramus and condyle on that side.

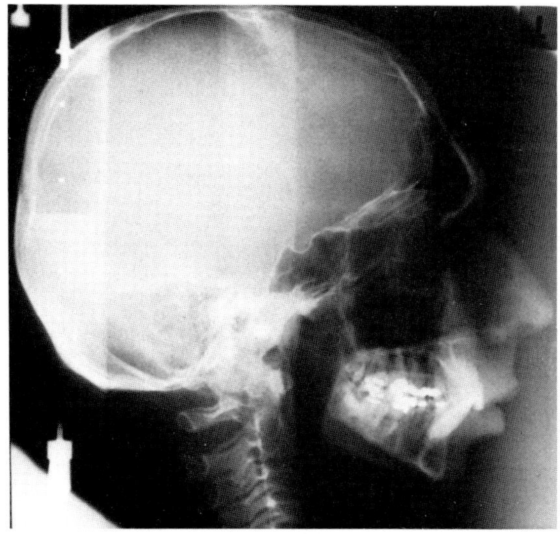

A

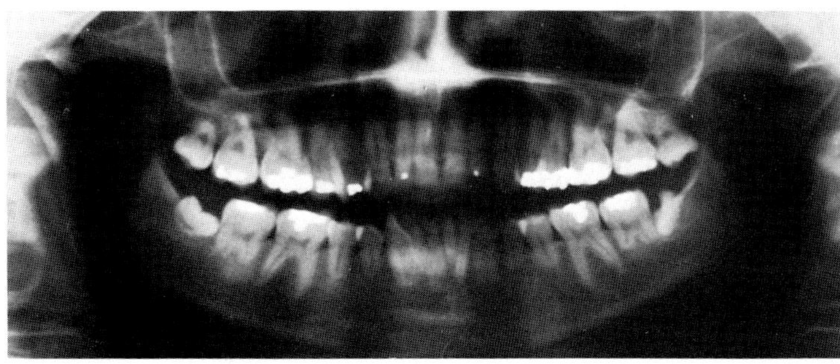

B

C

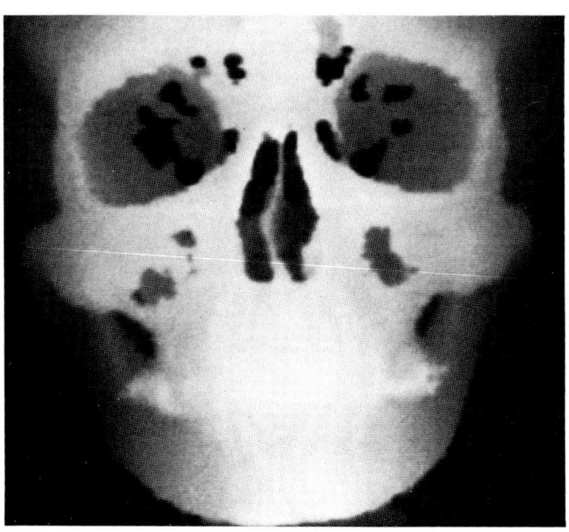

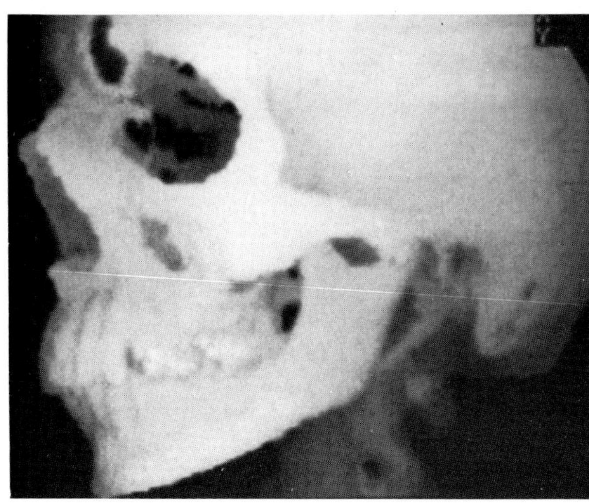

D

8

Tumors

Fibrous dysplasia, neurofibromatosis, and hemangiomas are conditions that produce tumors of great variety in the craniofacial region. With fibrous dysplasia there is expansion of the skeletal elements by an immature form of bone. Hemangiomas may cause underlying bony hypertrophy as a result of their hypervascular nature, but they may also be associated with bony erosion as a consequence of multiple expanding arteriovenous fistulae. Neurofibromas may also be vascular but tend to cause bony erosion.

Three-dimensional images are valuable for clearly defining the extent of the deformity of these conditions. However, the unpredictable modes of presentation make these tumors a significant imaging challenge. The low density substance of a fibrodysplastic mass may result in loss of image detail if routine thresholding is employed for the three-dimensional reconstruction. In these cases the three-dimensional images serve to complement existing modes of investigation, which should include two-dimensional computed tomography (CT) reformats and plain radiography. Similarly, the vascularity of hemangiomas and neurofibromas may produce secondary effects on the bony elements of the craniofacial skeleton, and these effects are well delineated with three-dimensional images. Although it is of particular value for the bony reconstruction phase of management and for the temporal plotting of bony distortion, three-dimensional imaging also serves as an adjunct for the traditional radiological techniques of angiography and two-dimensional computed tomography. More recently, magnetic resonance imaging has enhanced our understanding of the soft tissue limits of these tumors, and together with three-dimensional computed tomographic views it may provide the most complementary mode of imaging.

Fibrous Dysplasia

Fibrous dysplasia is a developmental anomaly of bone-forming mesenchyme. There are no obvious hereditary factors. It is characterized by the presence of fibrous connective tissue with a distinctive whorled pattern and trabeculae of immature nonlamellar bone. Of the benign tumors causing craniofacial deformity, fibrous dysplasia is one of those most frequently seen (Figs. 8.1–8.6). It is more common in female subjects and frequently presents during late childhood or early adolescence. It may be monostotic (Figs. 8.1–8.5) or polyostotic (Fig. 8.6) with skull involvement in 50% of cases. Cranial lesions may be entirely asymptomatic but progress slowly until adulthood with danger to such vital areas as the optic nerve (Figs. 8.1C–E and 8.6D–F) or middle ear structures. The frontal and sphenoidal bones are those most frequently involved (Figs. 8.1 and 8.2), but any skull bone may be affected, with symptoms dictated by the area involved (Figs. 8.3–8.5). The radiographic appearance depends on the proportion of bony and fibrous components. If the tumor is predominantly bony, there may be a ground-glass pattern or it may radiopaque. Involvement of the maxilla and base of the skull usually results in a radiopaque appearance (Figs. 8.2C and 8.3B).

Neurofibromatosis

Neurofibromatosis is a condition in which there is widespread hamartomatous overgrowth of the nerve sheath tissue. In 1882 von Recklinghausen described the syndrome of multiple neurofibromata, skin pigmentation, skeletal deformity, central nervous system involvement, and a predilection to malignancy (Figs. 8.7–8.9). The most common tumor of the syndrome is the neurofibroma involving the skin. It may be multiple and of varying size. Café au lait spots are the clinical hallmark of the disorder but are absent in nearly 10% of cases. In cases with craniofacial involvement there is a predilection for orbital structures (Figs. 8.7 and 8.8). There may be hypertrophy of skull bones with resultant asymmetry (Figs. 8.9G–I). Patients with neurofibromatosis may also have kyphoscoliosis, vertebral body involvement, limb or digital hypertrophy, bony cystic lesions, and an increased incidence of pheochromocytomas. The protean nature of the manifestations of neurofibromatosis precludes any simple classification of the disorder. It has autosomal dominant inheritance with variable penetrance and a mutation rate of approximately 50%.

Hemangiomas

Hemangiomas are local malformations of blood vessels. They may be classified, according to the predominant vessel involved, as arterial, venous, or capillary. Some involve all these vessels and may also have a lymphangiomatous component. Arterial hemangiomas progressively enlarge and compress surrounding tissues. Multiple feeding vessels contribute to their increased vascularity, providing abnormal pulsations and clinically detectable bruits. Venous hemangiomas are comprised of large blood lakes that can be reduced in size with digital compression only to slowly refill.

In the craniofacial region, venous hemangiomas with deep submucosal extensions into the orbit, pharynx, and neck may preclude surgical excision (Figs. 8.10 and 8.11). Hemangiomas that are predominantly capillary in composition range from the simple strawberry nevus, which undergoes spontaneous regression, to the more disfiguring port wine nevus, which persists throughout life. With Sturge-Weber syndrome (Fig. 8.12) a port wine nevus of the upper part of the face is associated with angiomatous changes in the leptomeninges of the ipsilateral cerebrum. Other features of the Sturge-Weber syndrome include a high incidence of seizure disorders (90%), mental retardation (30–50%), contralateral hemiparesis (30%), and glaucoma. Double contoured lines of calcification in the cerebral cortex are seen on computed tomography (Fig. 8.12C). The increased vascularity in the region of the hemangioma may be associated with underlying bone hypertrophy (Figs. 8.10C,D and 8.12D,E), or there may be bony erosion secondary to locally expanding vascular channels (Figs. 8.11D–F).

Recommended Reading

Altman NR, Altman DH, Wolfe SA, Morrison G: Three-dimensional CT reformation in children. AJR 146:1261, 1986.

Converse JM: Reconstructive Plastic Surgery. Saunders, Philadelphia, 1977.

Georgiade N, Masters F, Horton C: Ossifying fibroma (fibrous dysplasia) of the facial bones in children and adolescence. J Paediatr 46:36, 1955.

Jackson IT, Bite U: Three-dimensional computed tomographic scanning and major surgical reconstruction of the head and neck. Mayo Clin Proc 61:546, 1986.

Linder B, Campos M, Schafer M: CT and MRI of orbital abnormalities in neurofibromatosis and selected craniofacial anomalies. Radiol Clin North Am 25:787, 1987.

Spira M, Riccardi V: Neurofibromatosis. Clin Plast Surg 14:315, 1987.

Stal S, Hamilton S, Spira M: Hemangiomas, lymphangiomas and vascular malformations of the head and neck. Otolaryngol Clin North Am 19:769, 1986.

Toth BA, Ellis DS, Stewart WB: Computer-designed prostheses for orbitocranial reconstruction. Plast Reconstr Surg 81:315, 1988.

Van der Meulen J: Orbital neurofibromatosis. Clin Plast Surg 14:123, 1987.

Von Recklinghausen F: Über die multiplen Fibrome der Haut und ihre Beziehung zu den multiplen Neuromen. A. Hirschwald, Berlin, 1882.

A

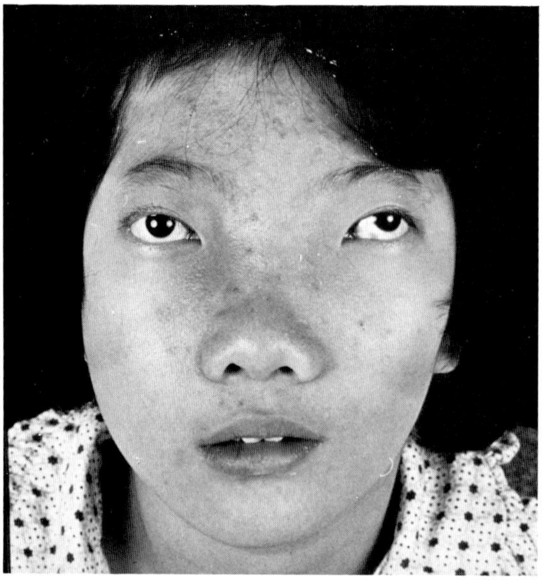

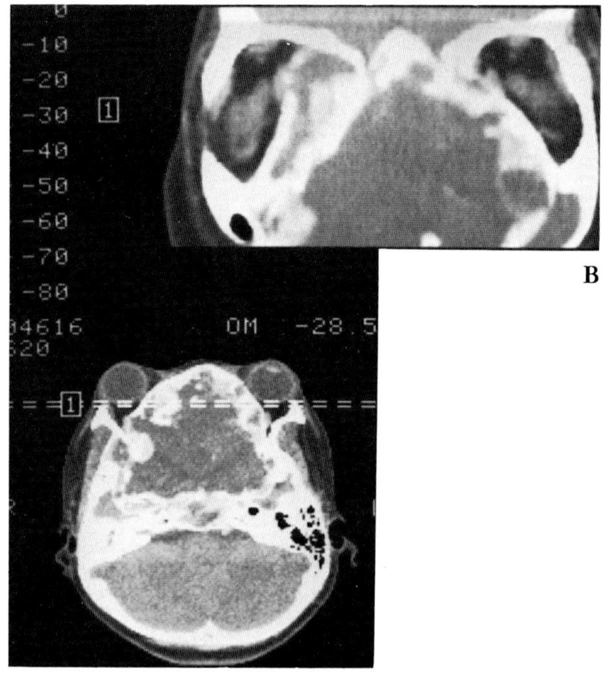

B

C

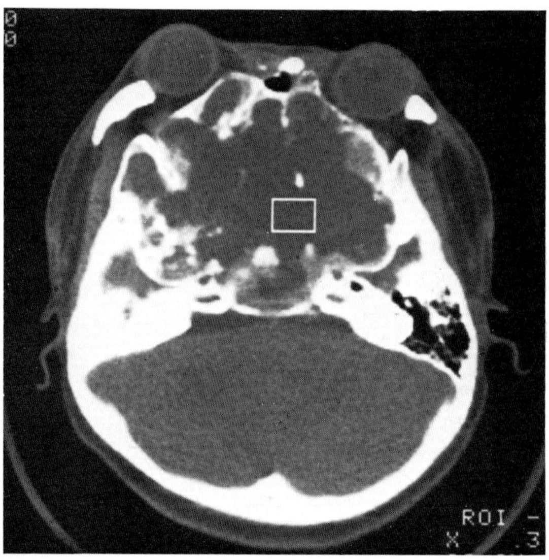

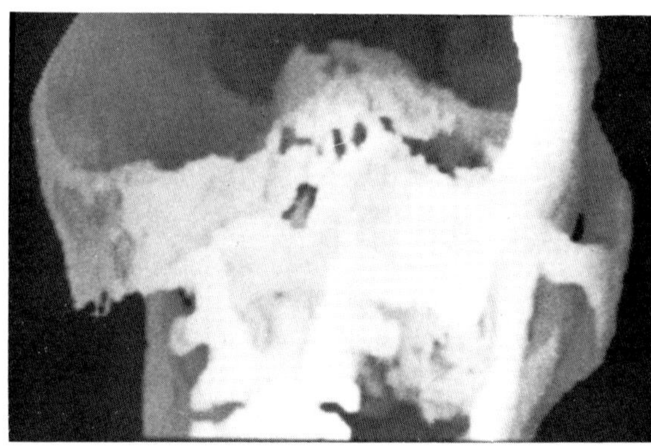

D

E

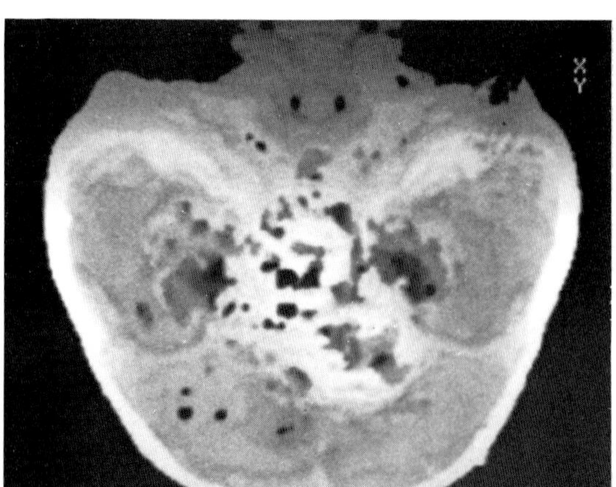

Fig. 8.1. A Gross hypertelorism resulting from skull base fibrous dysplasia. **B,C** Axial CT slices with coronal reconstruction show massive displacement of the globes by a lesion involving the anterior and middle cranial fossae. **D** Posterior view shows the lesion extending down through the base of the skull, medial to the right mandible. **E** Anterior fossa view shows the lesion extending throughout the anterior fossa and middle fossa.

A

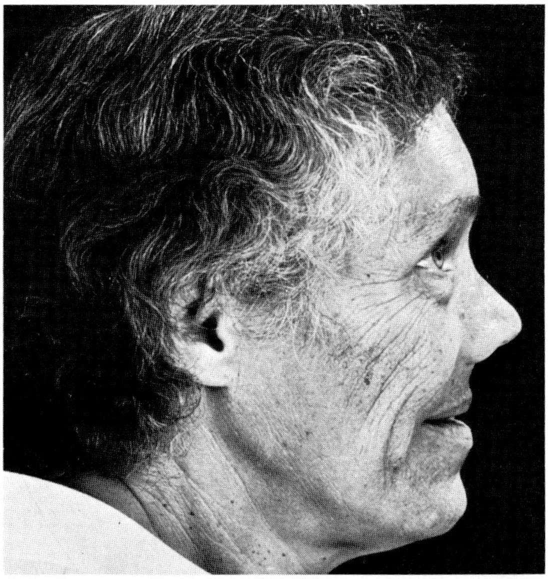

B

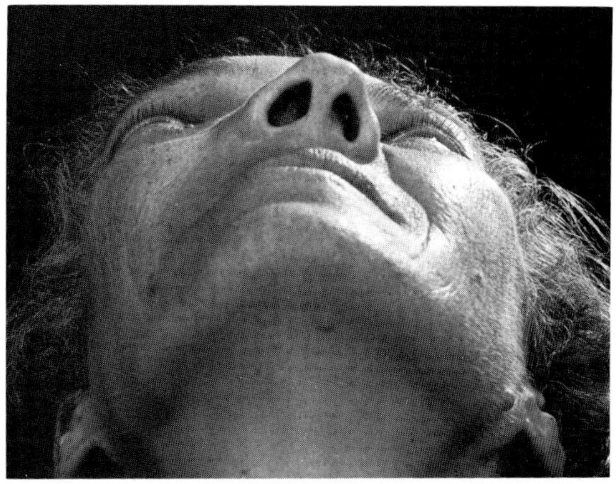

C

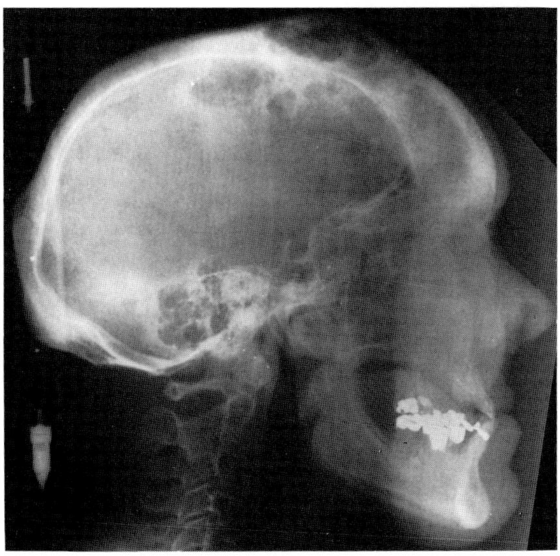

D

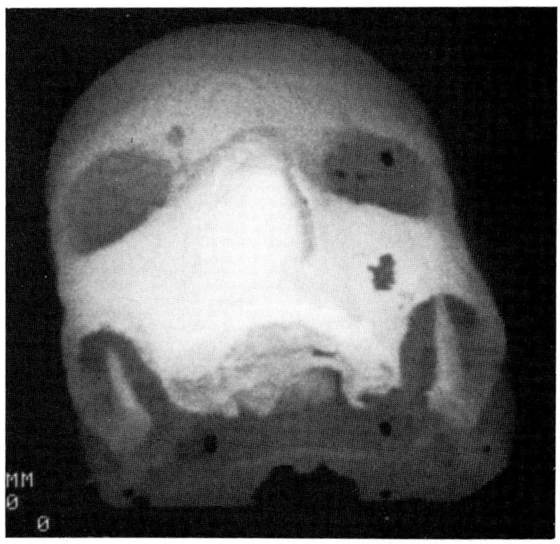

Fig. 8.2. A Middle-aged woman with acromegaly and fibrous dysplasia distorting the base of the skull, extending from the parietal region through the frontal region into the right orbit and maxilla. **B** Clinical view from below clearly shows the facial asymmetry. **C** Plain skull radiograph demonstrates the extent of the lesion from the parietal bone through to the frontal bone and entering the maxilla and postnasal space. **D** There is hypertelorism and outward rotation of the right orbit with obstruction of the nasal airway, which is reduced to a narrow slit on the left side of the fibrous dysplastic mass in the nose.

A B C D

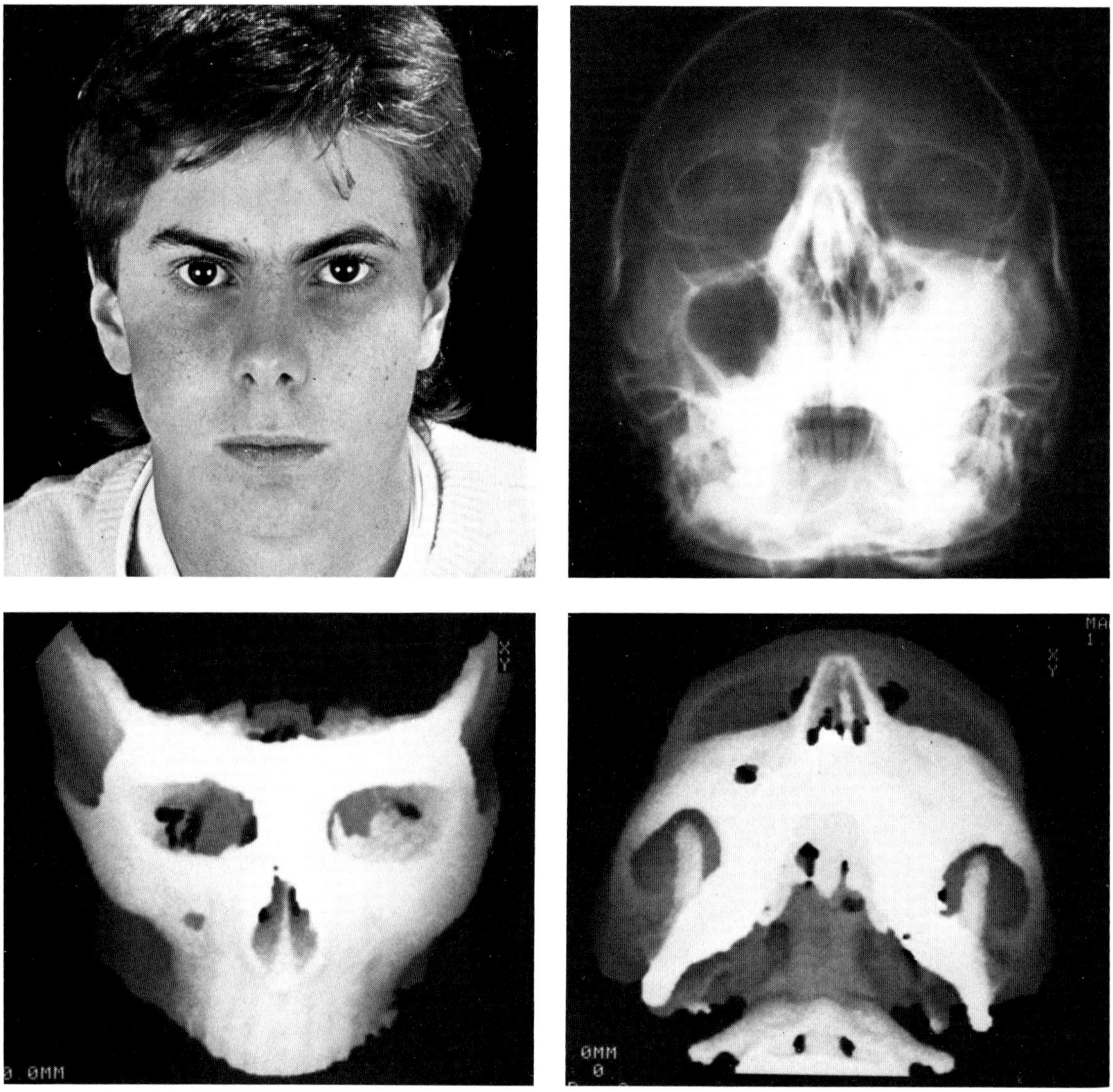

Fig. 8.3. A There may be minimal outward signs of maxillary fibrous dysplasia. **B** Characteristic ground-glass appearance of the fibrous dysplasia is seen in the region of the left maxilla. **C,D** There is expansion of the left maxilla and left zygomatic arch.

A B C

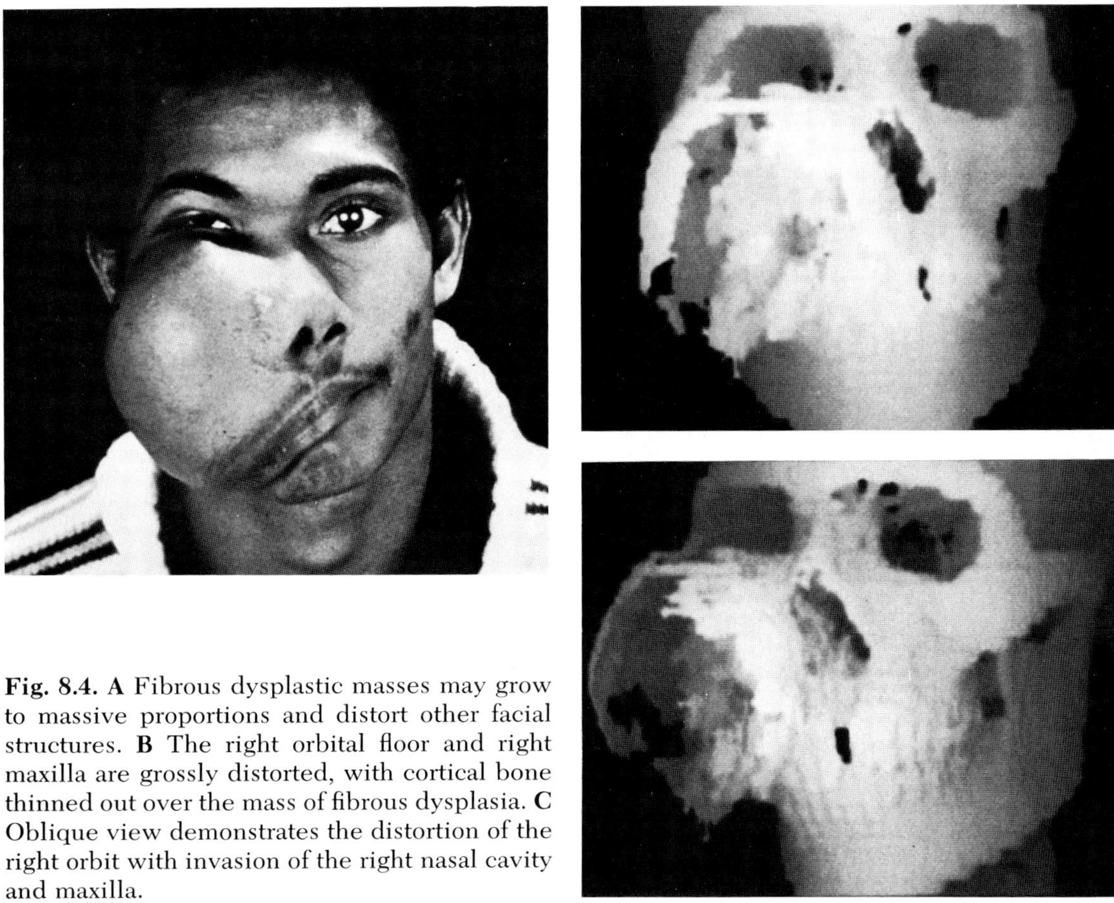

Fig. 8.4. A Fibrous dysplastic masses may grow to massive proportions and distort other facial structures. **B** The right orbital floor and right maxilla are grossly distorted, with cortical bone thinned out over the mass of fibrous dysplasia. **C** Oblique view demonstrates the distortion of the right orbit with invasion of the right nasal cavity and maxilla.

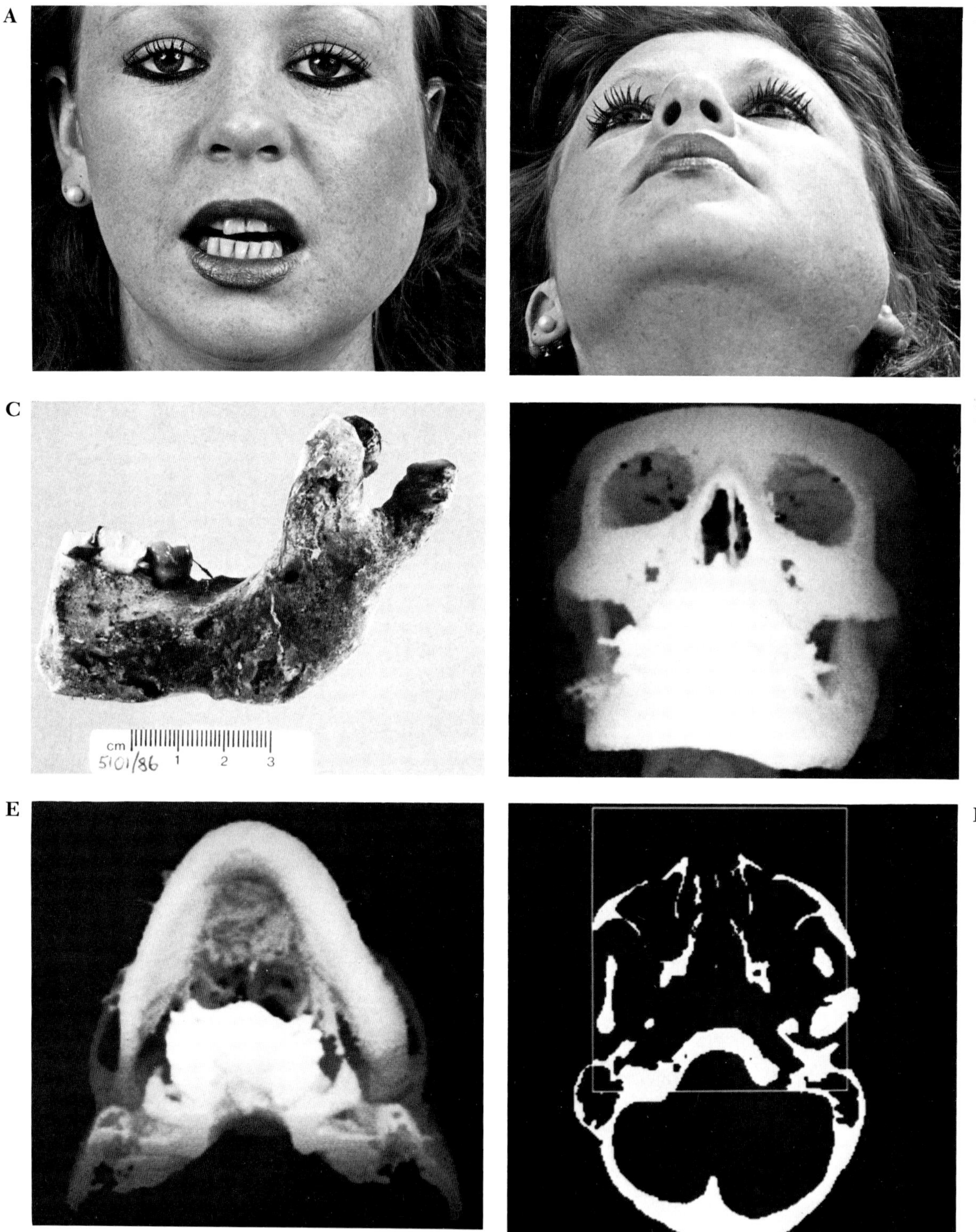
A
B
C
D
E
F
cm
5101/86 1 2 3

G

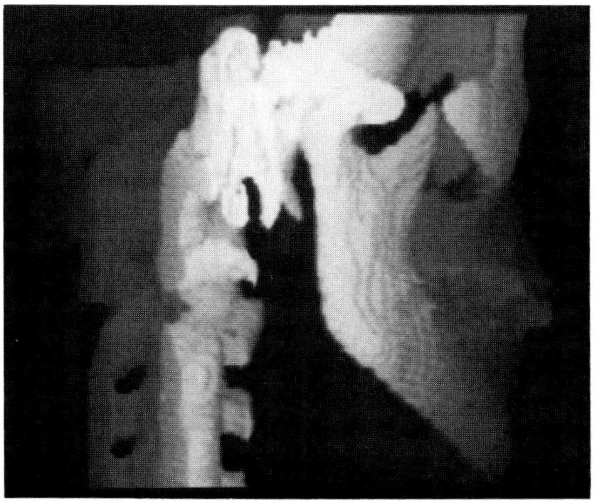

H

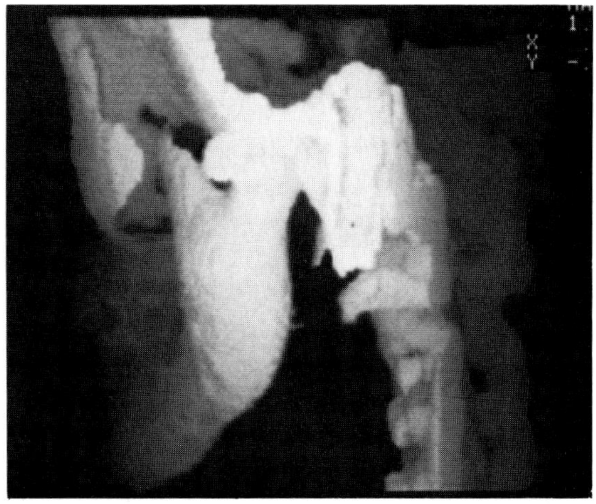

Fig. 8.5. A,B Fibrous dysplasia of the mandible has caused lower facial swelling on the left and malocclusion. **C** Resected operative specimen demonstrates the normal macroscopic appearance of fibrous dysplasia. **D** Fibrous dysplasia has invaded the left side of the mandible from the temporomandibular joint to the premolar region. **E** There is gross distortion of the temporomandibular joint on the left, and expansion of the mandible can be clearly seen in a basal view. **F** By predetermining an area of interest with a box cursor, selected structures can be viewed to the exclusion of others. In this case the mandible can be viewed without interference from the overlying zygoma. **G,H** Techniques described in Figure 8.5F have been used to compare normal and abnormal mandibular rami. The subregioned three-dimensional images of the mandibular rami are helpful for comparing the distorted side with the normal side.

A B

C D

E

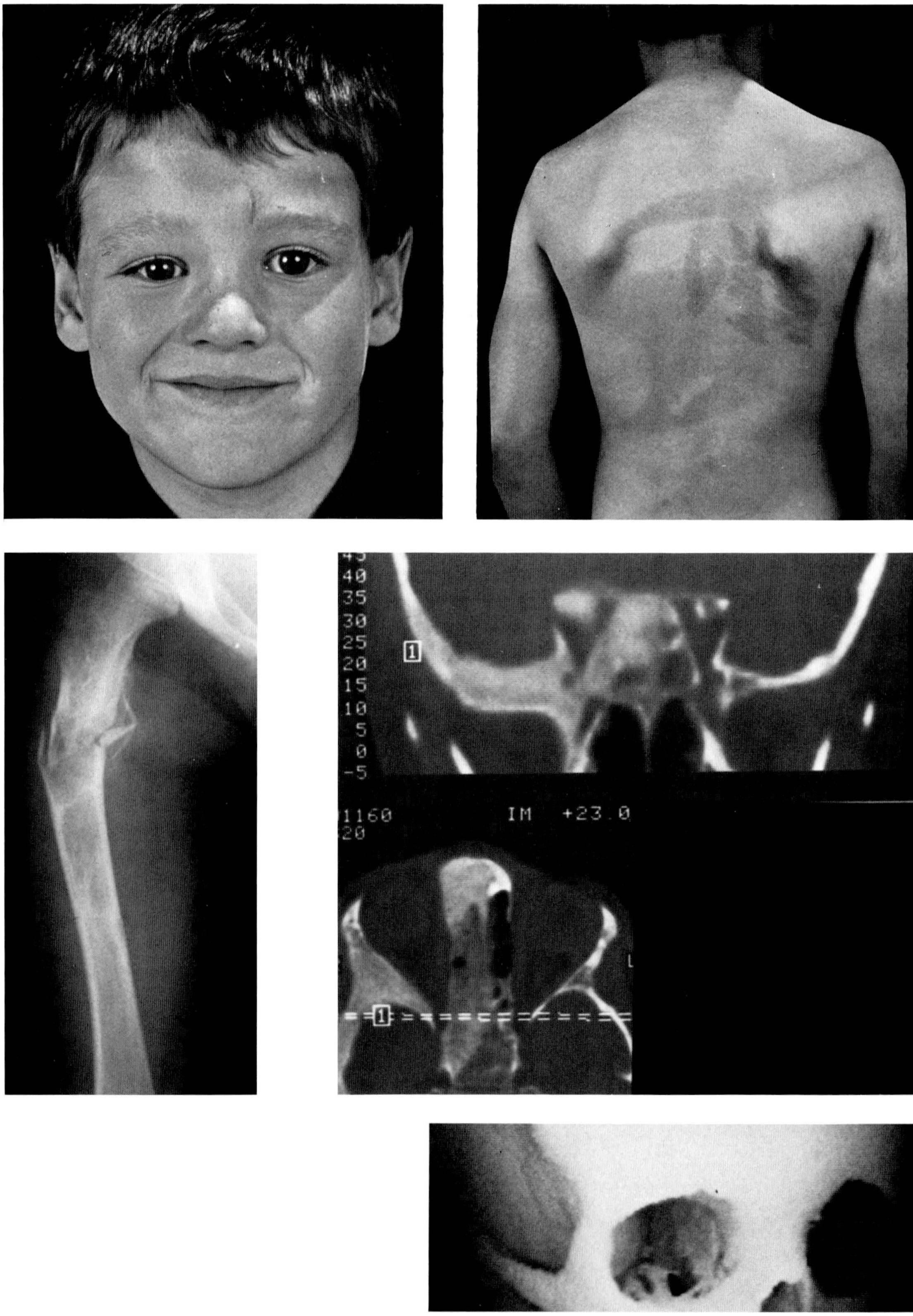

A

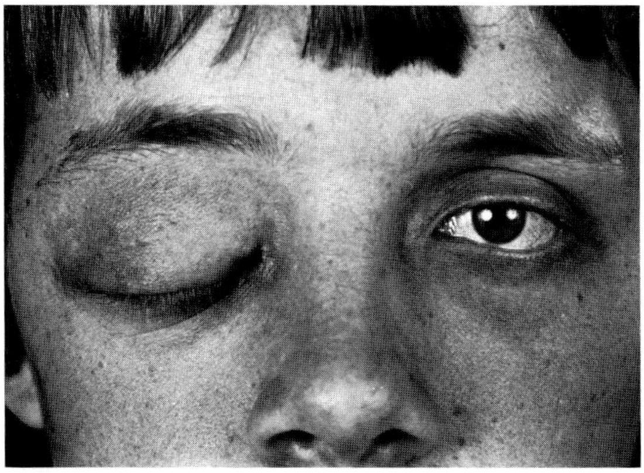

B

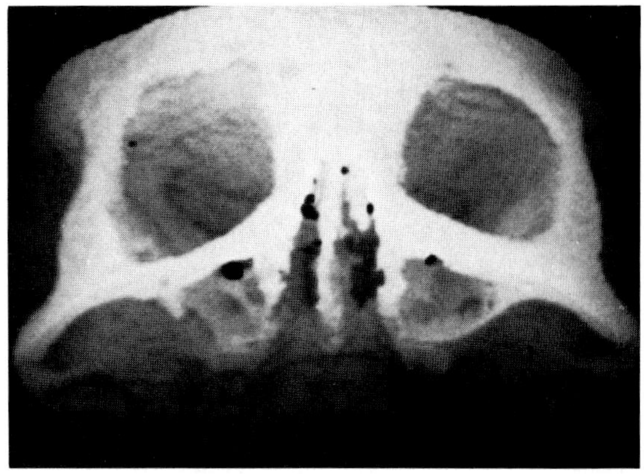

C

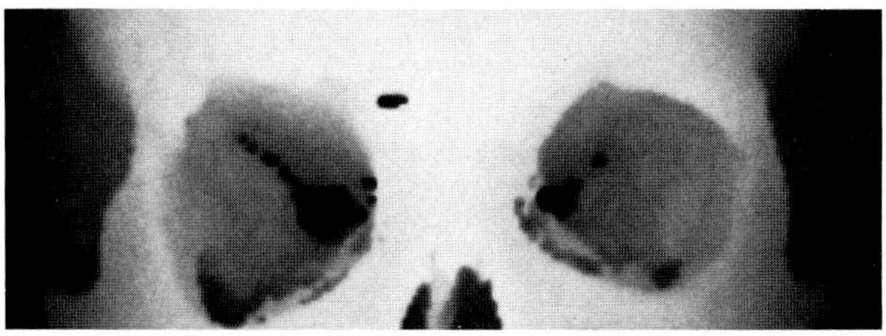

D

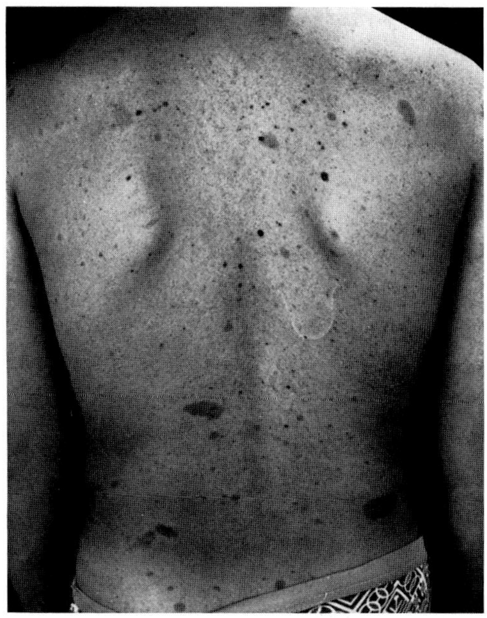

Fig. 8.7. A Neurofibromatosis with involvement of the right orbit and complete ptosis of the right upper eyelid. **B,C** Large right orbit with a depressed right infraorbital margin and orbital floor. **D** Typical multiple café au lait spots of neurofibromatosis are seen on the patient's back.

F

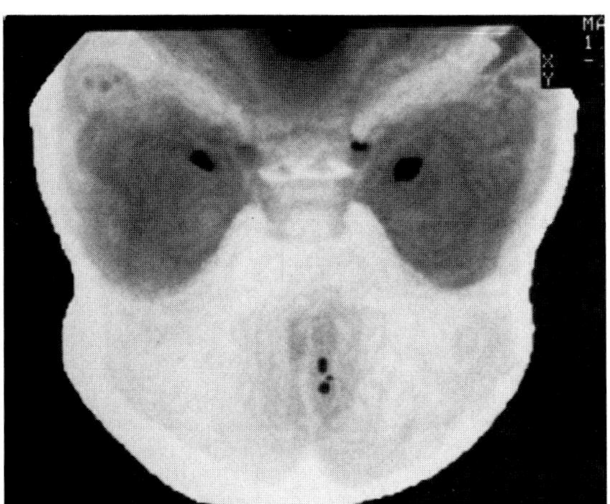

Fig. 8.6. A The craniofacial component of this patient's generalized fibrous dysplasia involves the right orbit. **B** View of the boy's back shows a café au lait spot, which is part of the syndrome. **C** Plain radiograph of this patient's right femur shows a fracture in an area of dysplastic bone. **D** Coronal CT reformatted image at the level of the optic canals demonstrates the fibrous dysplastic changes on the right. **E,F** The fibrous dysplastic changes are concentrated around the right orbit.

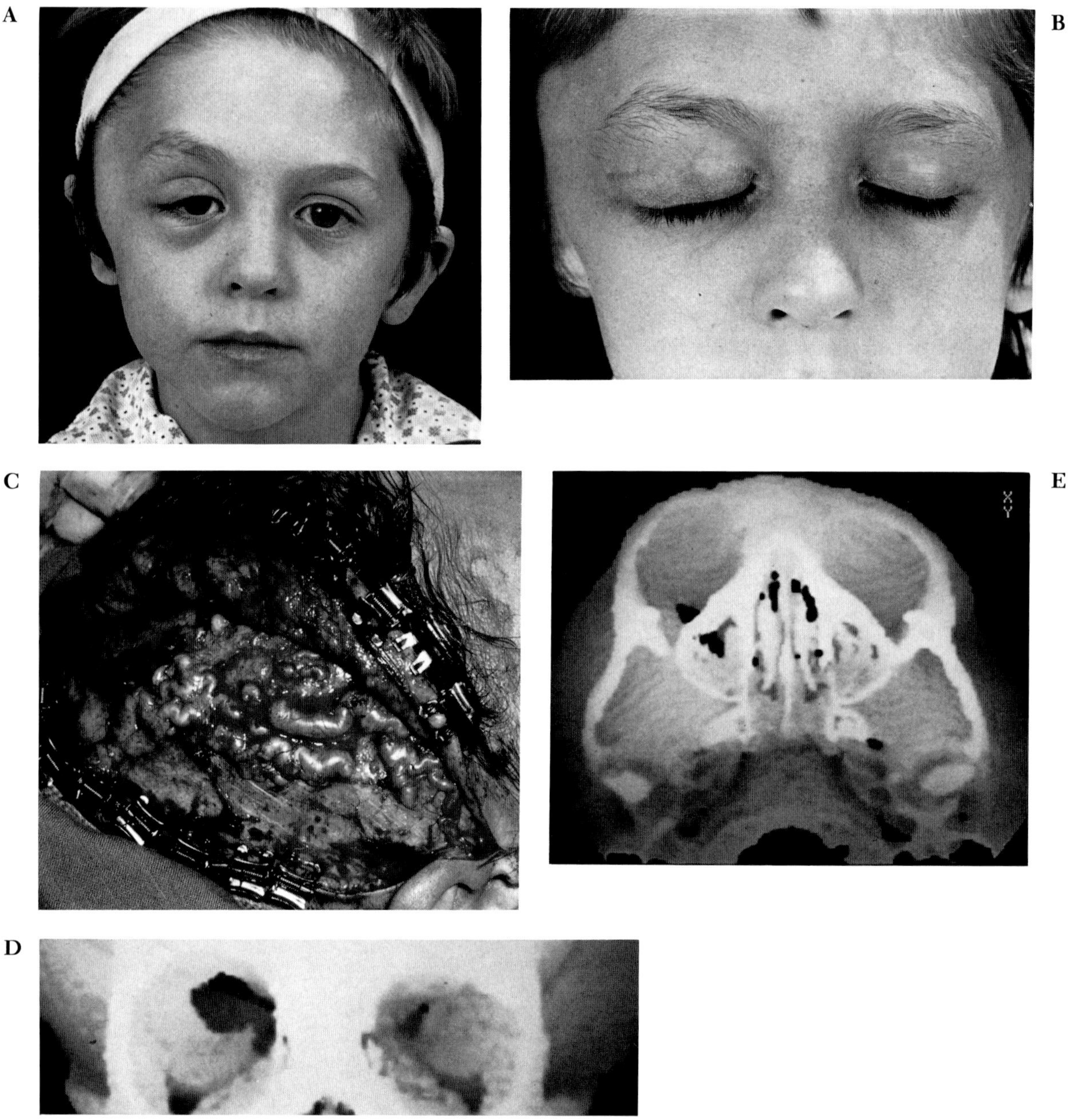

Fig. 8.8. **A** Orbital dystopia and ptosis secondary to a plexiform neurofibroma. **B** Right proptosis increases the prominence of the right upper eyelid. **C** Operative view of a large plexiform neurofibroma following the course of the scalp veins. **D** Right orbit is expanded, and there is erosion of the sphenoid. **E** Vertical expansion of the right orbit is evident when both sides are compared from below.

A

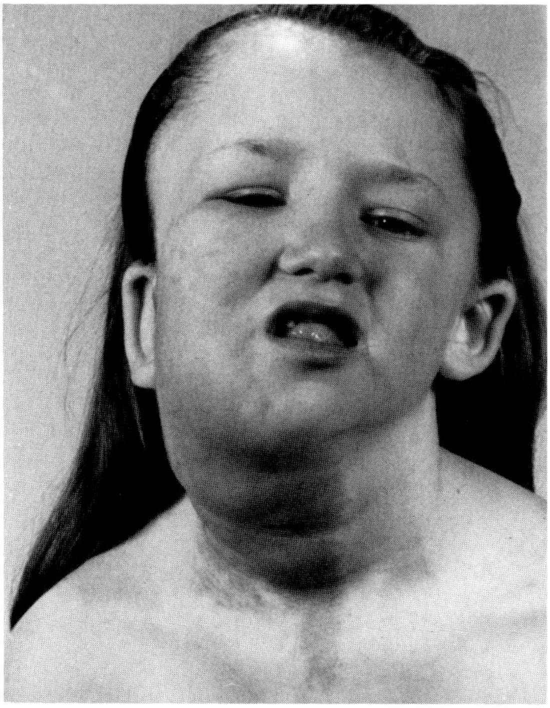

B

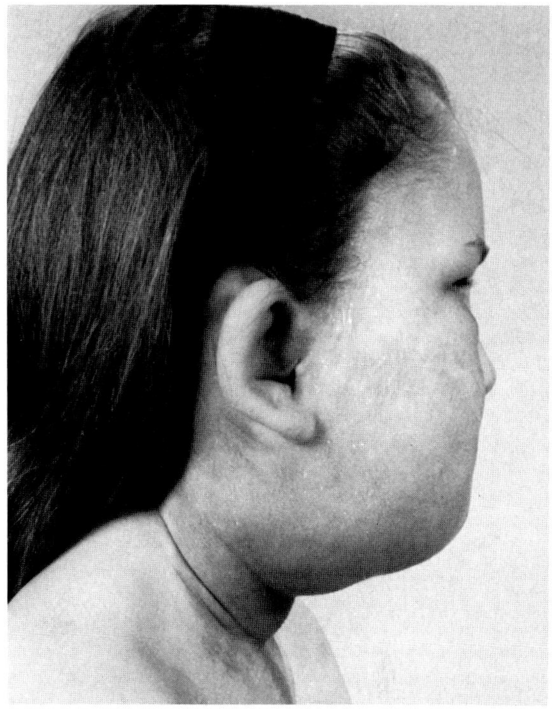

C

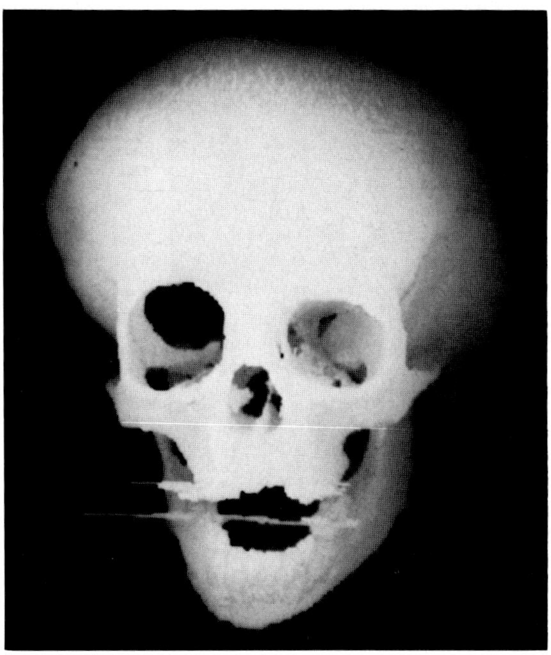

D

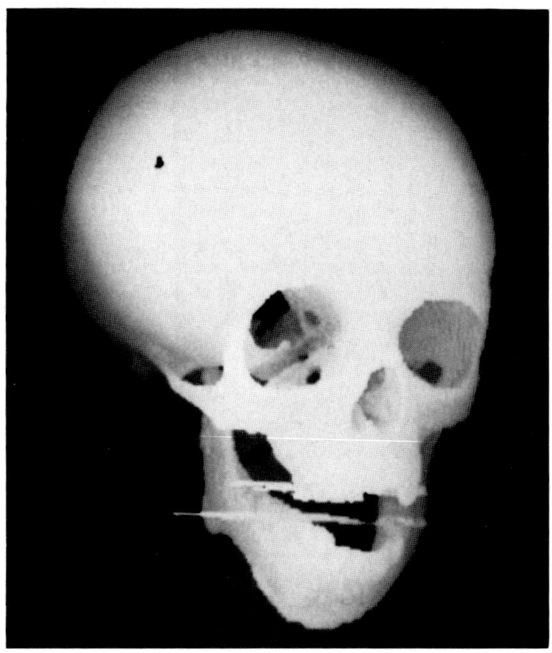

Fig. 8.9. **A** Gross facial distortion as a result of neurofibromatosis. Note the pigmented cervical skin. **B** Lateral view of patient in Figure 8.9A. **C** Orbital involvement by the neurofibroma causes marked expansion of the volume of the right orbit. Horizontal streaking is the result of dental restorations. **D** Erosion of the right sphenoid provides direct communication of the orbital and cranial cavities. **E-I** See pp. 124 and 125.

E F G H

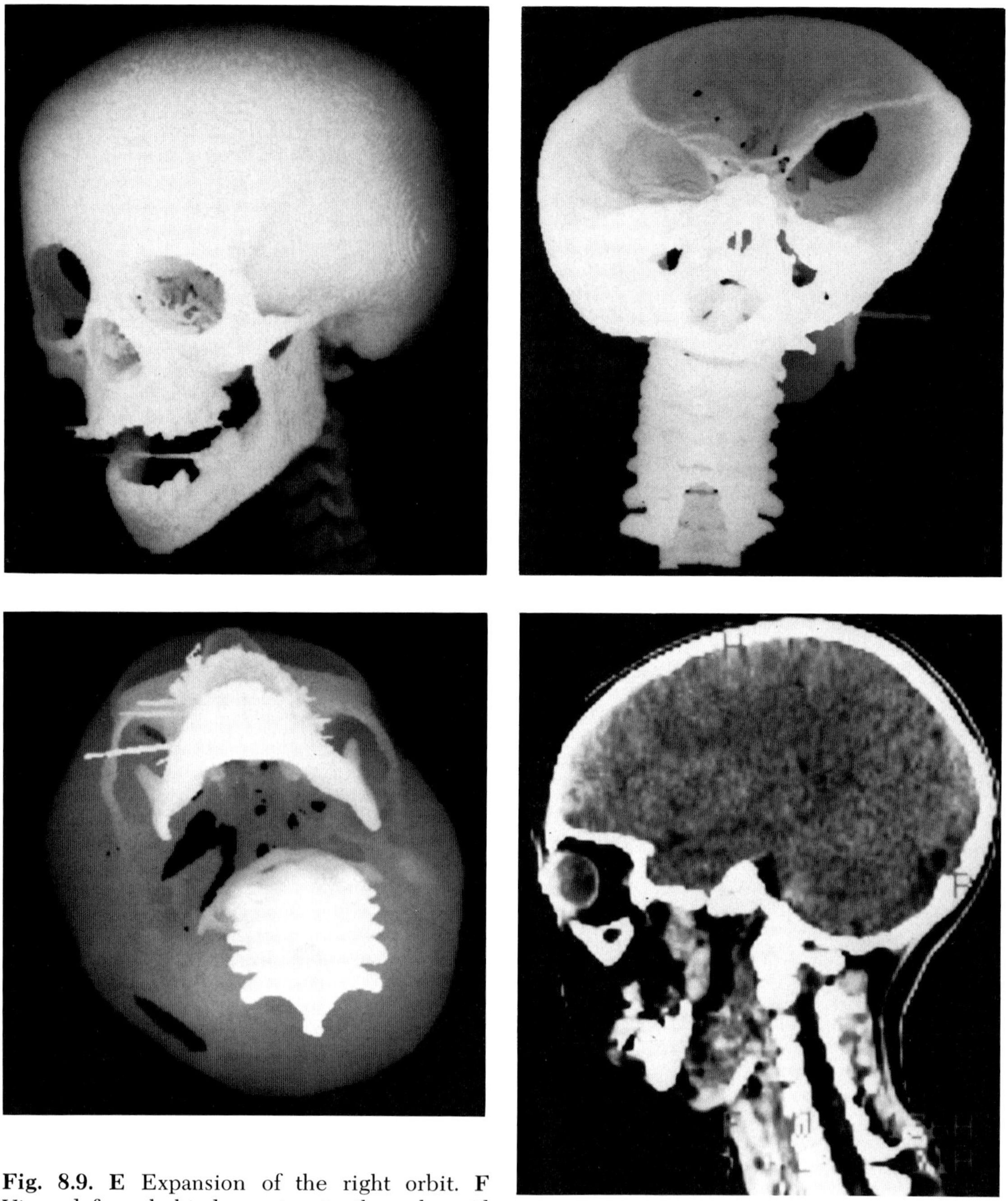

Fig. 8.9. E Expansion of the right orbit. **F** Viewed from behind, erosion in the sphenoid bone is obvious. **G** Hemicranial asymmetry. **H** Left midpupillary sagittal reformatted image from data acquired for three-dimensional imaging. **I** Right midpupillary reformat. Note the posterior orbital defect that resulted from sphenoidal erosion. Observe the recessive temporal lobe surrounded by cerebrospinal fluid. Also note that the right pupil is enophthalmic.

A

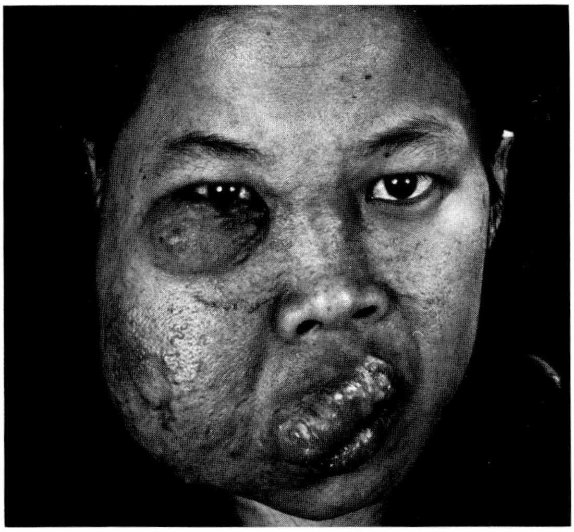

B

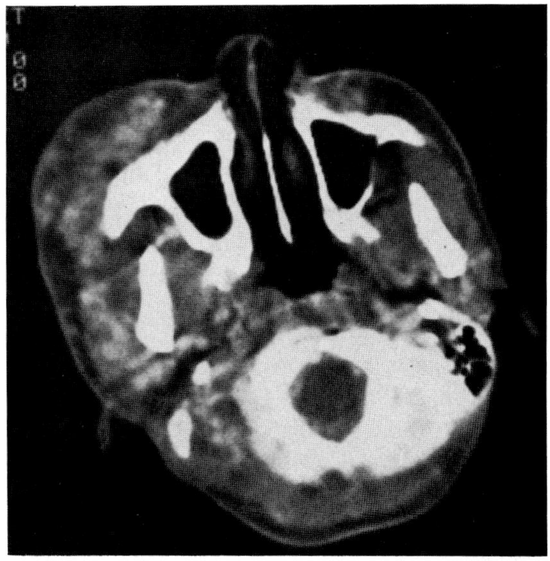

C

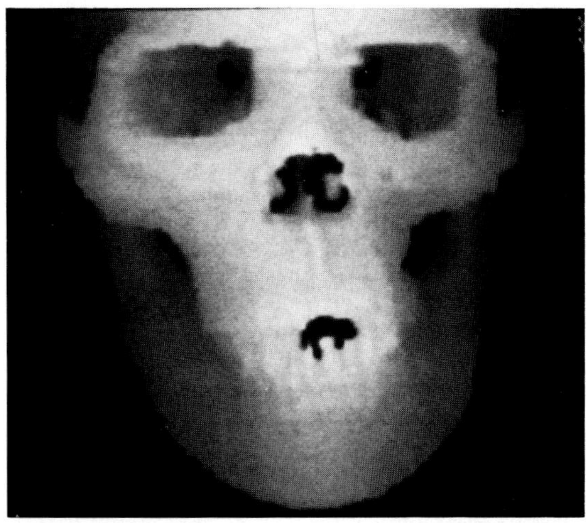

D

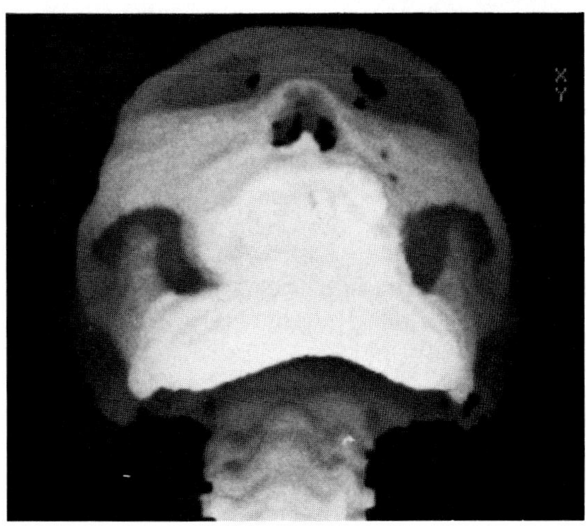

Fig. 8.10. A Large facial hemangiomas may cause distortion of external features but may also have deep extensions. In this patient the vascular mass extended from the skull base and orbit through to the maxilla and mandible. **B** The relation between soft tissue and the underlying bony deformity can be seen on the axial CT scan. **C** Bone in close proximity to the hemangioma may undergo hypertrophy. There is enlargement of the right zygoma, right maxilla, and right side of the mandible. **D** Chin-up view indicates the increased bone size on the right side.

I

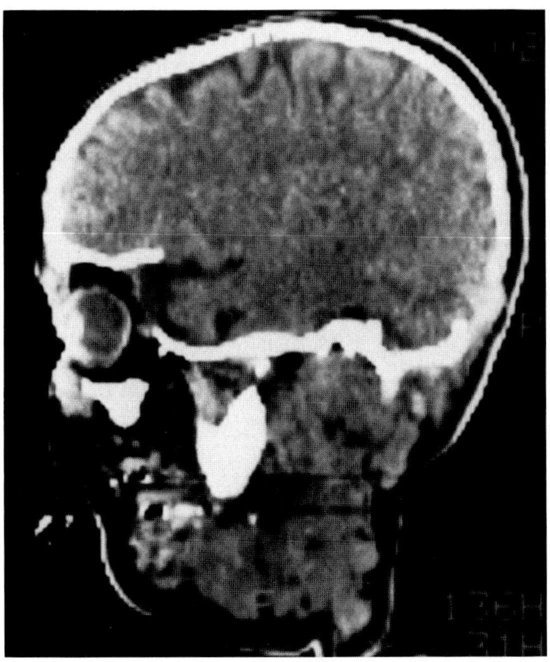

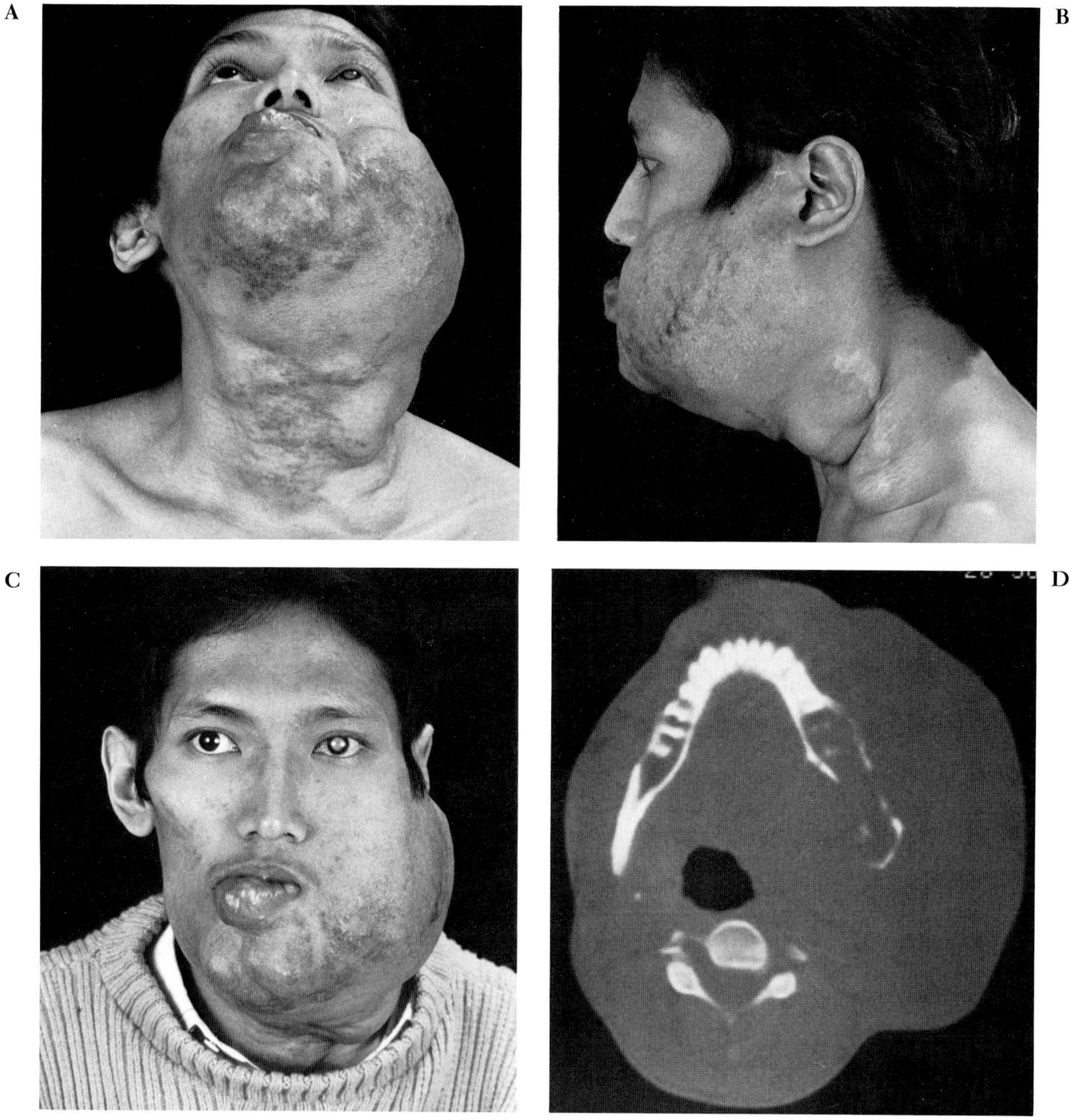

Fig. 8.11. A–C Massive hemangioma involving the neck and face. **D** Axial CT image at the level of the mandible. Note the extensive expansion of the soft tissue by the hemangioma. The mandibular body has been eroded by the arteriovenous connections of the hemangioma. **E,F** Mandibular distortion is well visualized with three-dimensional imaging. At operation the lower border was papyraceous and traversed by huge vascular channels.

E F

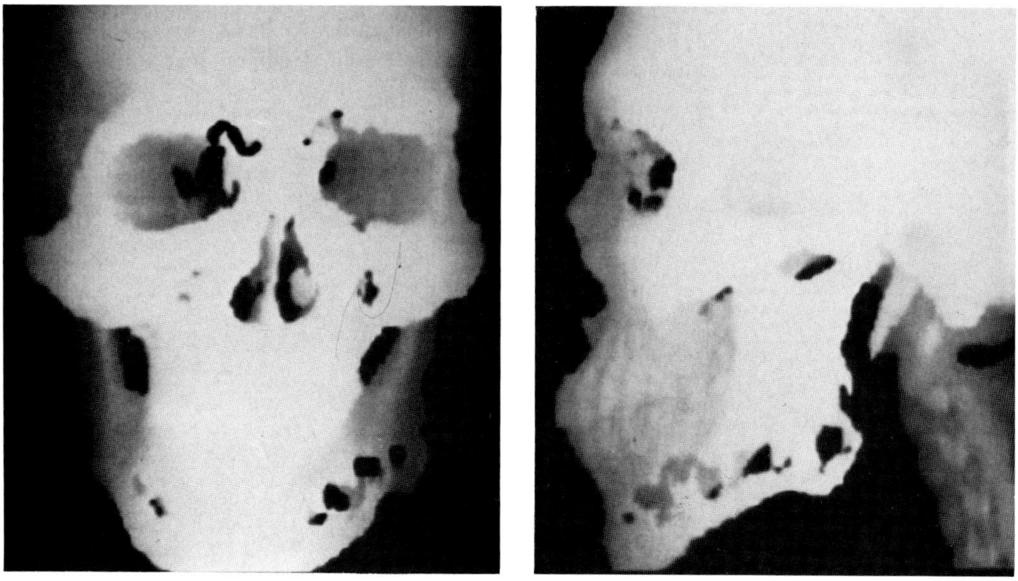

Fig. 8.11 (contd)

A

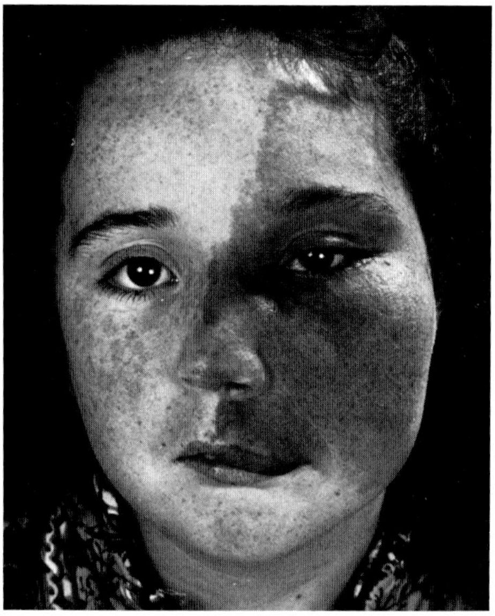

B

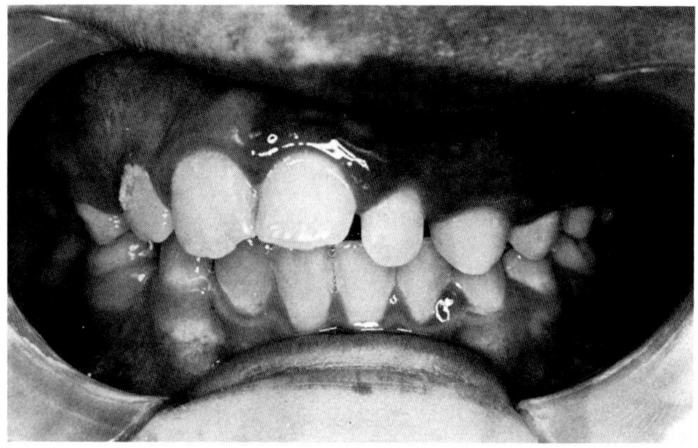

C

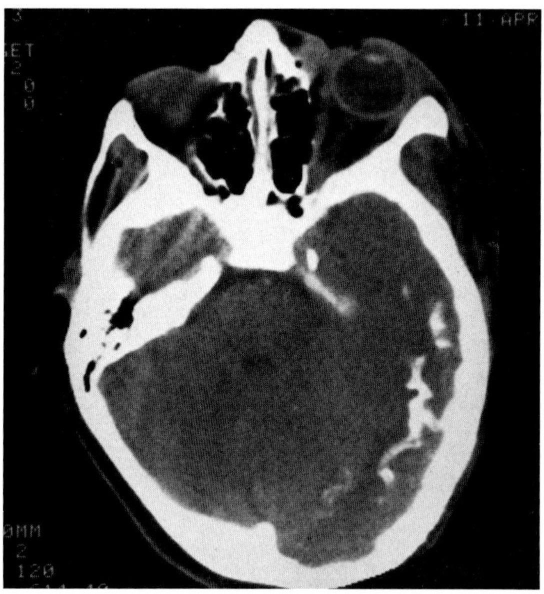

D

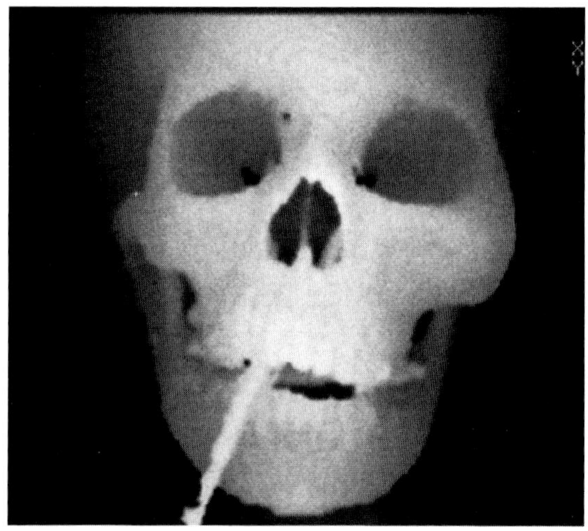

E

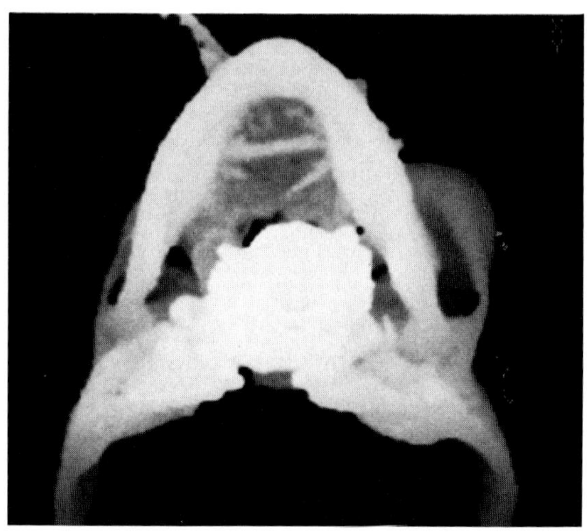

Fig. 8.12. A Typical distribution of the capillary hemangioma of Sturge-Weber syndrome is over the cutaneous areas of the first and second divisions of the trigeminal nerve. **B** Dentoalveolar view shows extension of the hemangioma onto the left maxillary alveolus. **C** Intracranial changes with this syndrome may include tramline calcifications as shown on axial CT scans. **D** Increased size of the left zygoma and maxilla are clearly demonstrated on the three-dimensional image. **E** Basal view confirms the bony distortion by demonstrating the abnormal protuberance of the left zygoma and deviation of the chin point.

9

Trauma

In 1901 Rene Le Fort recognized the possibility of improving fracture diagnosis by understanding the common fracture pathways. Le Fort relied on dissections of impacted cadavers to define the fracture patterns sustained by the human face after relatively low velocity impact. Throughout the 20th century, however, there has been a steady increase in the velocity of impacts to the craniofacial region as well as improved ability to image fractures. Plain radiography has been extensively employed, and a number of views have been described to reduce the problem of overlapping images from the complex three-dimensional anatomy of the craniofacial region.

Although many other imaging modalities have been described for the diagnosis of craniofacial trauma, computed tomography (CT) now plays an essential role. For delineation of a fracture pathway through the three-dimensional anatomy of the craniofacial skeleton, three-dimensional CT images are invaluable, as they overcome the need for subjective mental reconstructions of a large number of two-dimensional images. These three-dimensional CT reconstructions clearly demonstrate the distorted spatial relations of severely disrupted bones within the craniofacial skeleton, although fractures with only minor degrees of displacement are not well identified.

Orbitocranial Fractures

Complex fractures may be accurately assessed from three-dimensional reformatted images following CT scanning (Figs. 9.1–9.5). The pattern of the cranial component of the fracture may be classified as:

Transfrontal (Figs. 9.1C and 9.2C,D)
Transorbital (Figs. 9.2C, 9.3A,B, 9.4B, and 9.5A,B)
Transbasal
  Transethmoidal (Fig. 9.2E)
  Transsphenoidal (Fig. 9.3C)

Midfacial Fractures

René Le Fort (1869–1951) described three varieties of fracture involving the middle one-third of the face.

Le Fort I (Guerin) Fracture

The Le Fort I fracture (Figs. 9.6) is a horizontal fracture traversing the maxilla above the alveolar process and extending through the lower one-third of the nasal septum and inferior portion of the maxillary sinuses (Fig. 9.6C–E). It crosses the pterygomaxillary fissures and the pterygoid plates in their lower one-thirds. The result is a mobile segment containing the palate, maxillary alveolar process, portions of the palatine bones, and lower one-third of the pterygoid plates.

Le Fort II (Pyramidal) Fracture

The Le Fort II (pyramidal) fracture (Fig. 9.7) radiates in an inferior direction from the nasal bridge and crosses the medial wall of the orbit, skirting the infraorbital foramen to run adjacent to the zygomaticomaxillary suture (Figs. 9.7C,D). It then extends posteriorly along the lateral wall of the maxilla, crossing the pterygoid plates at a higher level than a Le Fort I fracture. The mobile bony segment formed is pyramidal in shape and contains most of the maxilla.

Le Fort III Fracture (Craniofacial Disjunction)

The Le Fort III fracture (Figs. 9.8 and 9.9) is the most severe midface fracture. It results from the bones of the middle one-third of the facial skeleton being forced backward and downward along the sloping cranial base, thus separating the whole of the midfacial skeleton from the cranial base. The fracture extends posteriorly, initially horizontally from the frontonasal suture through the ethmoid bone toward the apex of the orbit and passing below the optic foramen to reach the pterygomaxillary fissure. The fracture crosses the lateral orbital wall to the zygomaticofrontal suture and separates the greater wing of the sphenoid and the zygoma. The zygomatic arch is usually fractured adjacent to the zygomaticotemporal suture. The fracture extends downward and backward across the sphenopalatine fossa to disrupt the root of the pterygoid plates. The mobile segment consists of the maxilla and the midfacial bones with which it articulates.

Gunshot Wounds

Severe bone and soft tissue disruption may result from close range gunshot injury (Figs. 9.10 and 9.11). The extent of injury depends on the mass, velocity, and shape of the missile(s). Three-dimensional images clearly depict the extent of bone disruption.

Old Trauma

Despite the prevalence of craniomaxillofacial surgical centers and techniques, patients still present with uncorrected craniofacial fractures and persistent malalignment after ineffective treatment (Figs. 9.12–9.15). Images obtained after late presentation of craniofacial trauma are affected by the healing process (the formation of callus, remodeling, and new bone formation). The fracture lines are often less clear, and the healing process often distorts the original pattern of the fracture.

Recommended Reading

Cooper PW, Kassel EE, Gruss JS: High resolution CT scanning of facial trauma. AJNR 4:495, 1983.

Cooter RD, David DJ: Computer-based coding of fractures in the craniofacial region. Br J Plast Surg 42:17, 1989.

David DJ: New perspectives in the management of severe craniofacial deformity. Ann Coll Surg Engl 66:270, 1983.

Gillespie JE, Isherwood I, Barker GR, Quayle AA: Three-dimensional reformations of computed tomography in the assessment of facial trauma. Clin Radiol 38:523, 1987.

Gruss JS: Naso-ethmoid-orbital fractures: classification and role of primary bone grafting. Plast Reconstr Surg 75:303, 1985.

Halimi P, Doyon D, Bekkali F, Idir ABC: Contribution of computerized tomography to the radiological study of craniofacial injuries. J Neuroradiol 13:253, 1986.

Koltal PJ, Wood GW: Three-dimensional CT reconstruction for the evaluation and surgical planning of facial fractures. Otolaryngology 95:10, 1986.

Le Fort R: Etude expérimentale sur les fractures de la machoire supérieure. Rev Chir Paris 23:208, 360, 479, 1901.

Merville L: Multiple dislocations of the facial skeleton. J Maxillofac Surg 2:187, 1974.
Rowe JL, Williams JL: Maxillofacial Injuries. Vol 1–11. Churchill Livingstone, New York, 1985.
Tessier P: The scope and principles, dangers and limitations, and the need for special training in orbitocranial surgery. In: Transactions of the Fifth International Congress of Plastic and Reconstructive Surgery. Butterworth, Melbourne, 1971.

A B C D

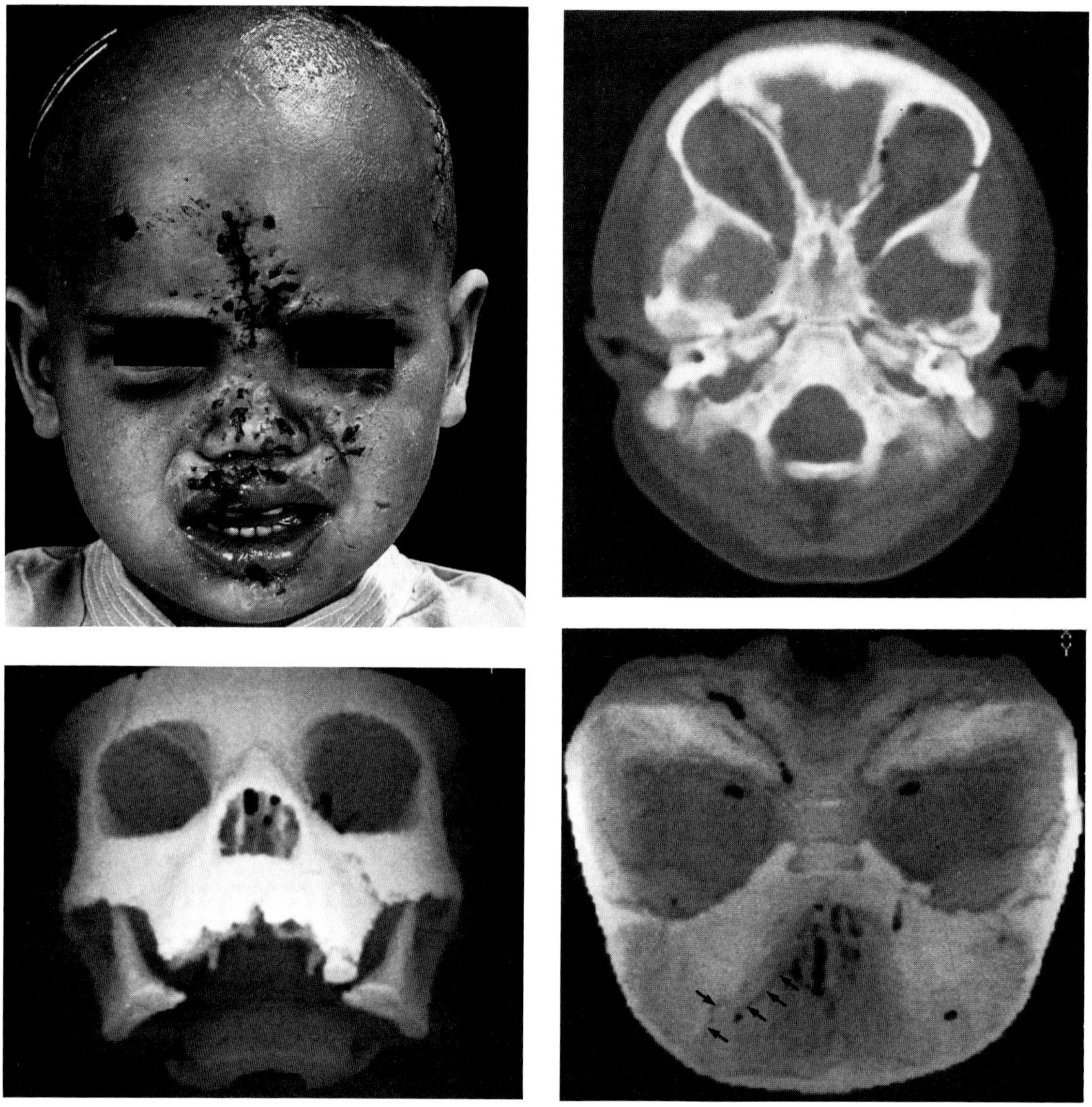

Fig. 9.1. A Postoperative view of the lacerations sustained by a patient involved in a motor vehicle accident. **B** Fractures of the anterior skull are evident. **C** One fracture extends from the right supraorbital margin into the frontal bone. There is also a fracture of the left zygomaticomaxillary junction. **D** Undisplaced fracture is seen extending from the right supraorbital rim to the posterior limit of the cribriform plate.

A

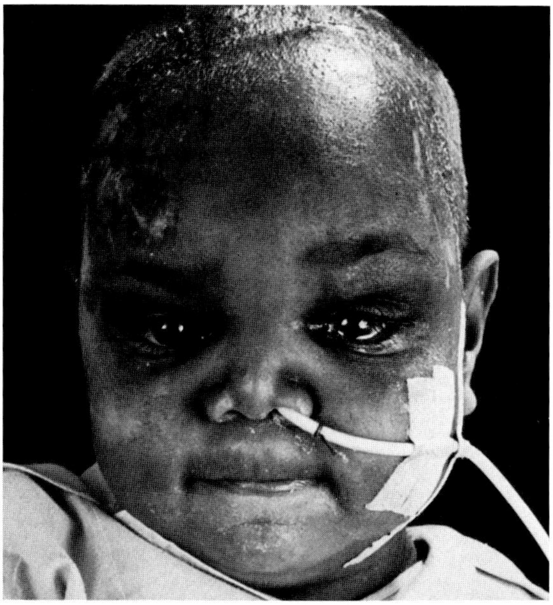

B

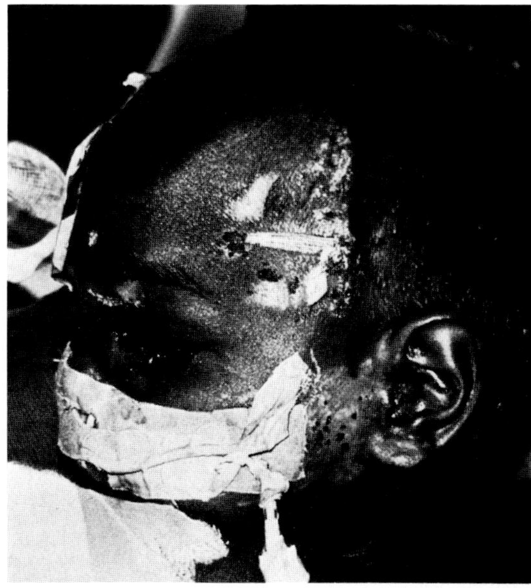

C

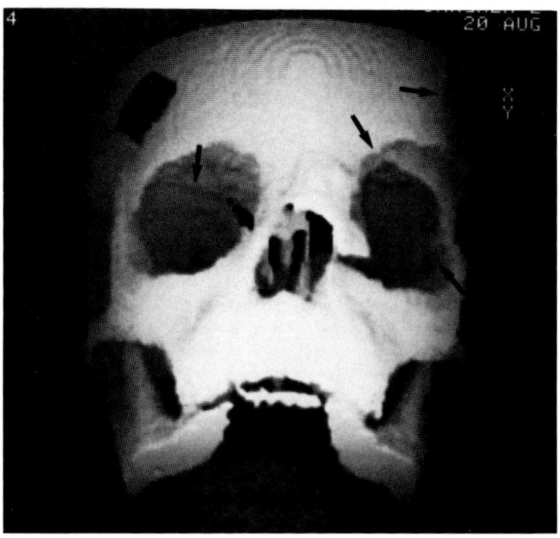

D

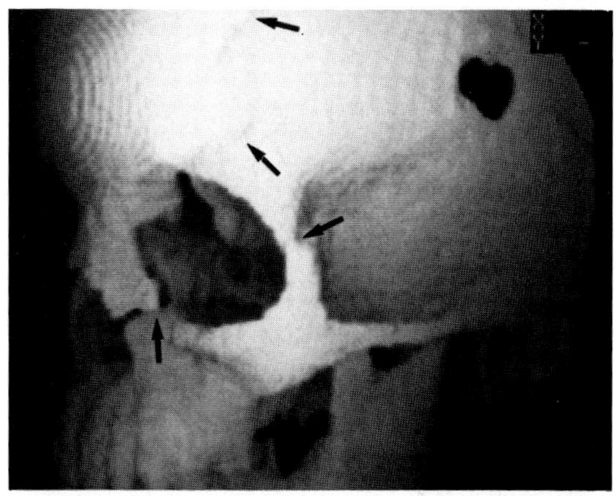

E

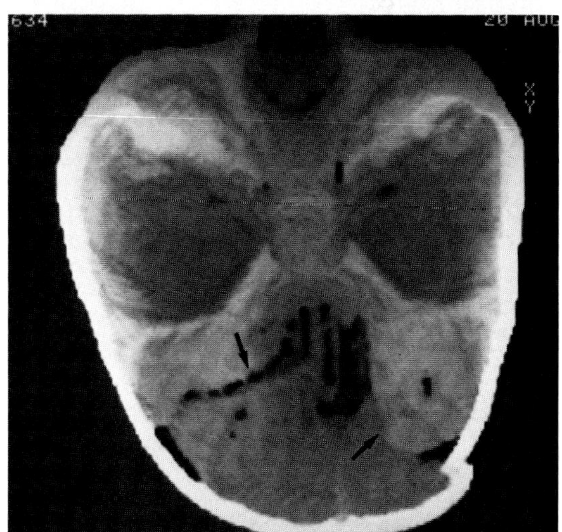

Fig. 9.2. A,B Young Aboriginal boy who was run over by a vehicle had minimal soft tissue trauma compared with the severe nature of his craniofacial fractures. **C** The pattern of fractures is demonstrated on the osseous image. **D** The fracture extends from the frontal bone crossing the supraorbital margin to traverse the nasoethmoidal complex. There is complete disruption of the frontozygomatic suture. Also note a surgical burr hole in the parietal region. **E** The fracture crosses the floor of the anterior fossa, involving the cribriform plate.

A

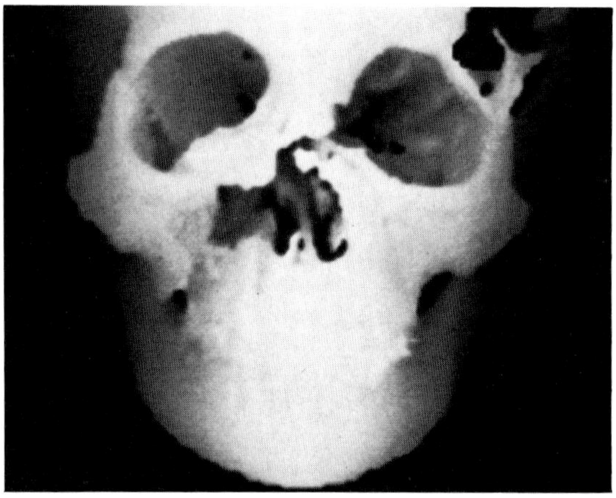

B

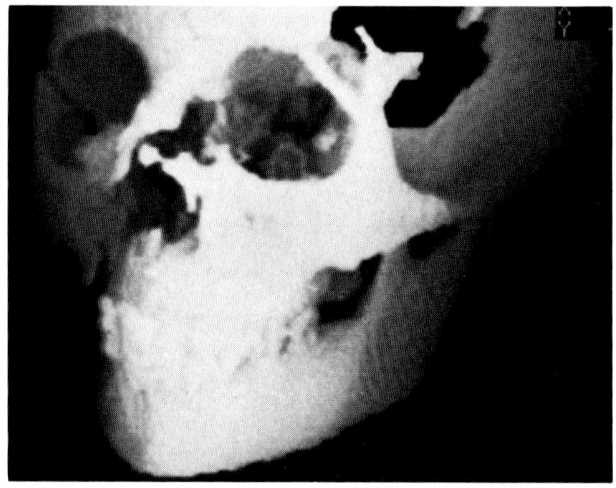

C

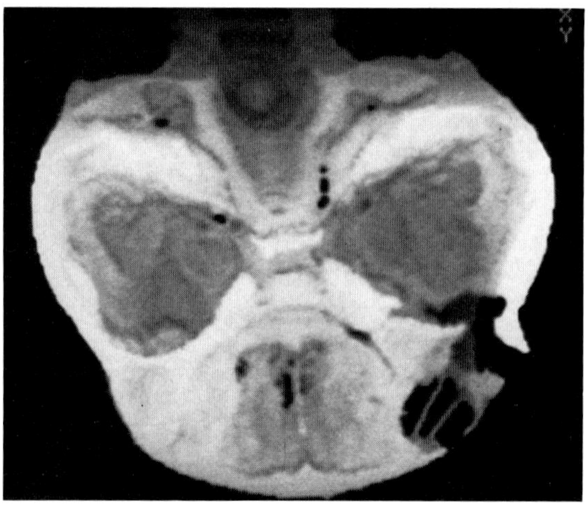

Fig. 9.3. A Bony disruption extends from the left frontal region across the facial structures to involve the right zygoma, which is laterally displaced. There is a Le Fort I fracture extending from the nasal aperture on the right. **B** The extent of traumatic bone loss is clearly depicted on the oblique view. **C** Three-dimensional image scanning is a useful radiographic technique for defining the skull base extension of fractures. This patient's fracture transversed the sphenoid bone and entered the middle cranial fossa.

A B C

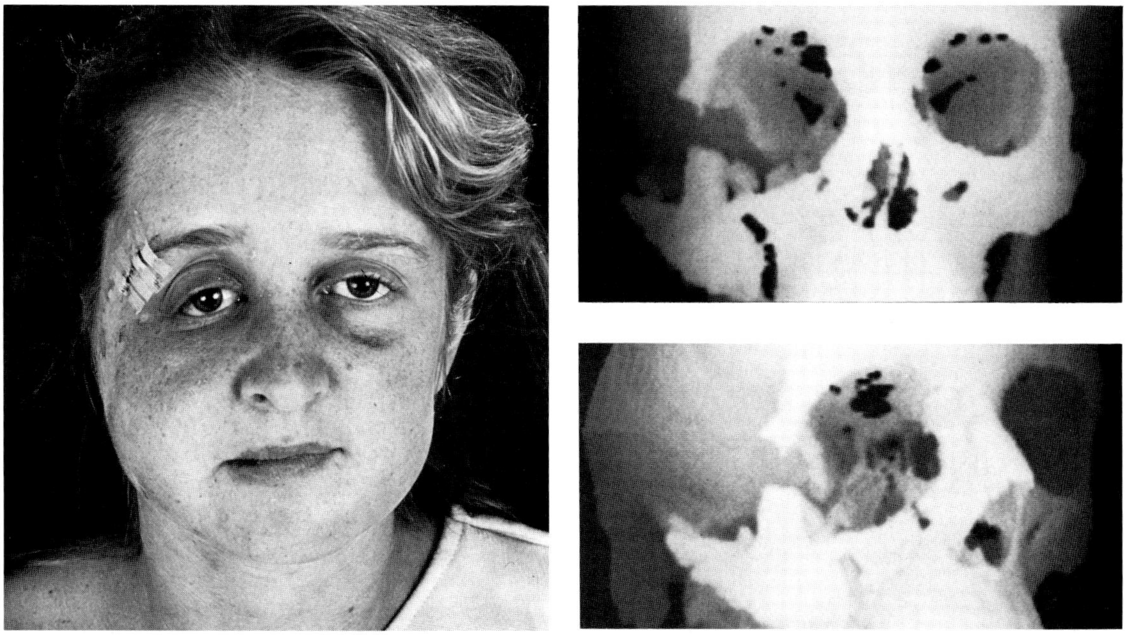

Fig. 9.4. A Orbital dystopia and flattening of the right cheek resulted from a severe fracture after this girl was trodden on by a horse. B Inferolateral displacement of the right zygomatic complex had increased the orbital volume, and there is further disruption of the inferior orbital margin medially. C The individual bony fragments are most clearly seen with a variety of views. The zygomatic complex is divided into a large lateral fragment and a smaller medial fragment.

A B

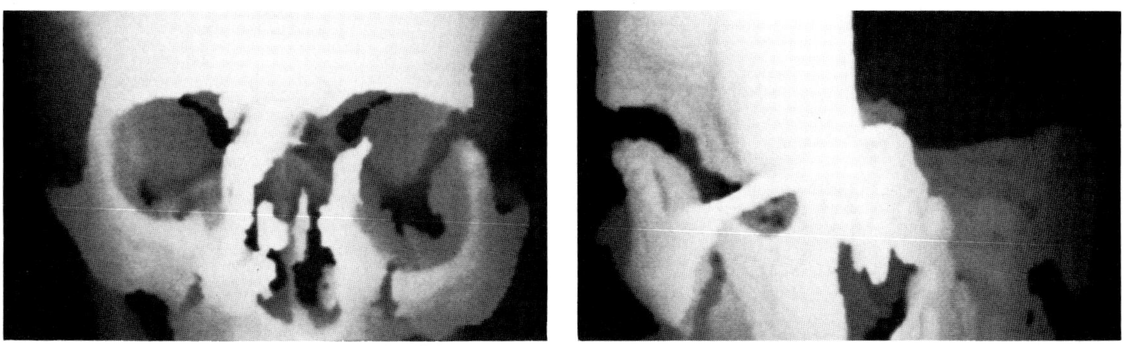

Fig. 9.5. A There is disruption of the left orbit with downward and outward displacement of the zygomatic complex. The vertical component of a Le Fort II fracture is seen through the right maxilla. B Posterior views are useful for demonstrating the relation between the displaced fragment and the frontal bone.

A B C D E

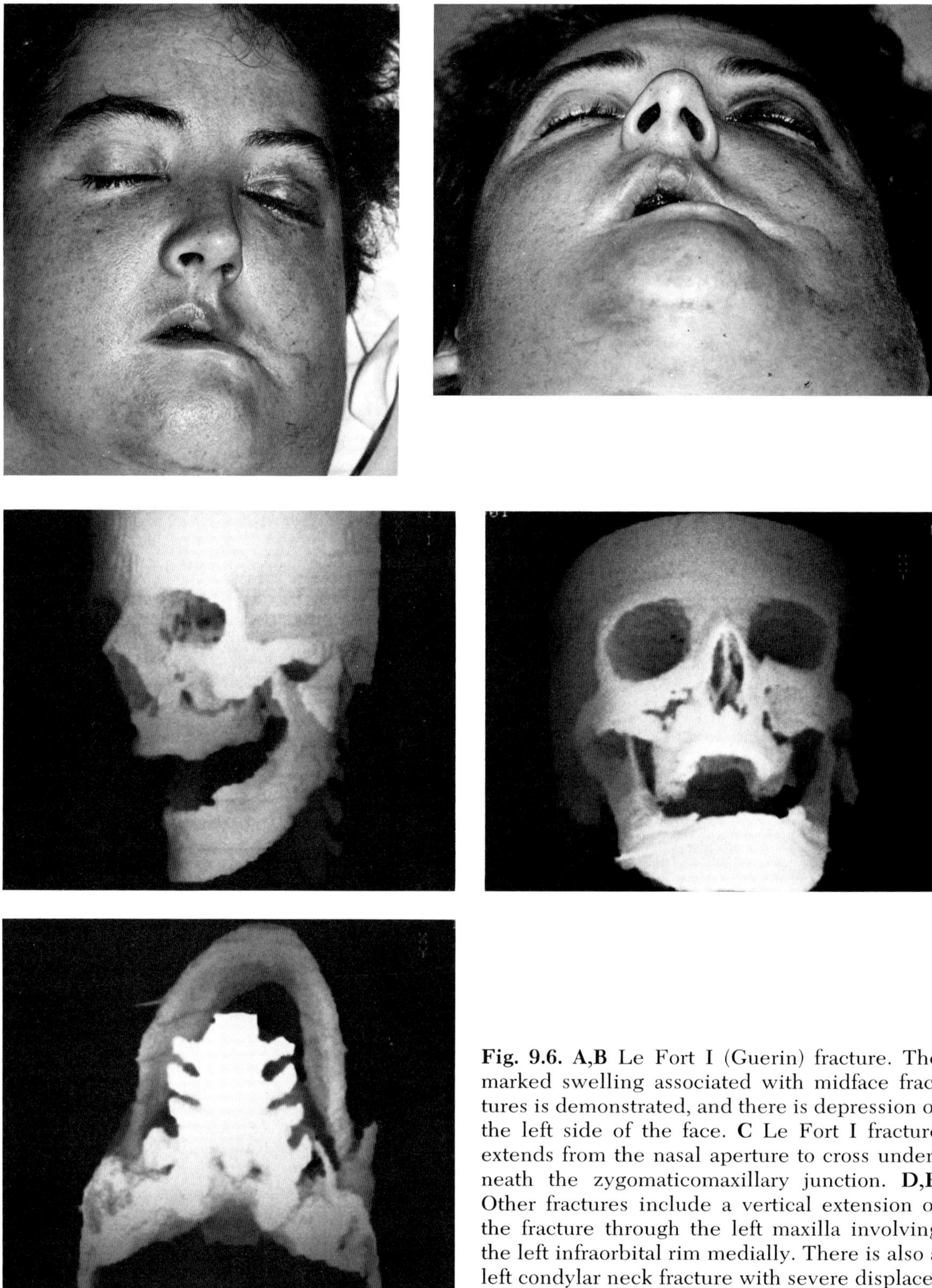

Fig. 9.6. A,B Le Fort I (Guerin) fracture. The marked swelling associated with midface fractures is demonstrated, and there is depression of the left side of the face. **C** Le Fort I fracture extends from the nasal aperture to cross underneath the zygomaticomaxillary junction. **D,E** Other fractures include a vertical extension of the fracture through the left maxilla involving the left infraorbital rim medially. There is also a left condylar neck fracture with severe displacement.

A B C D

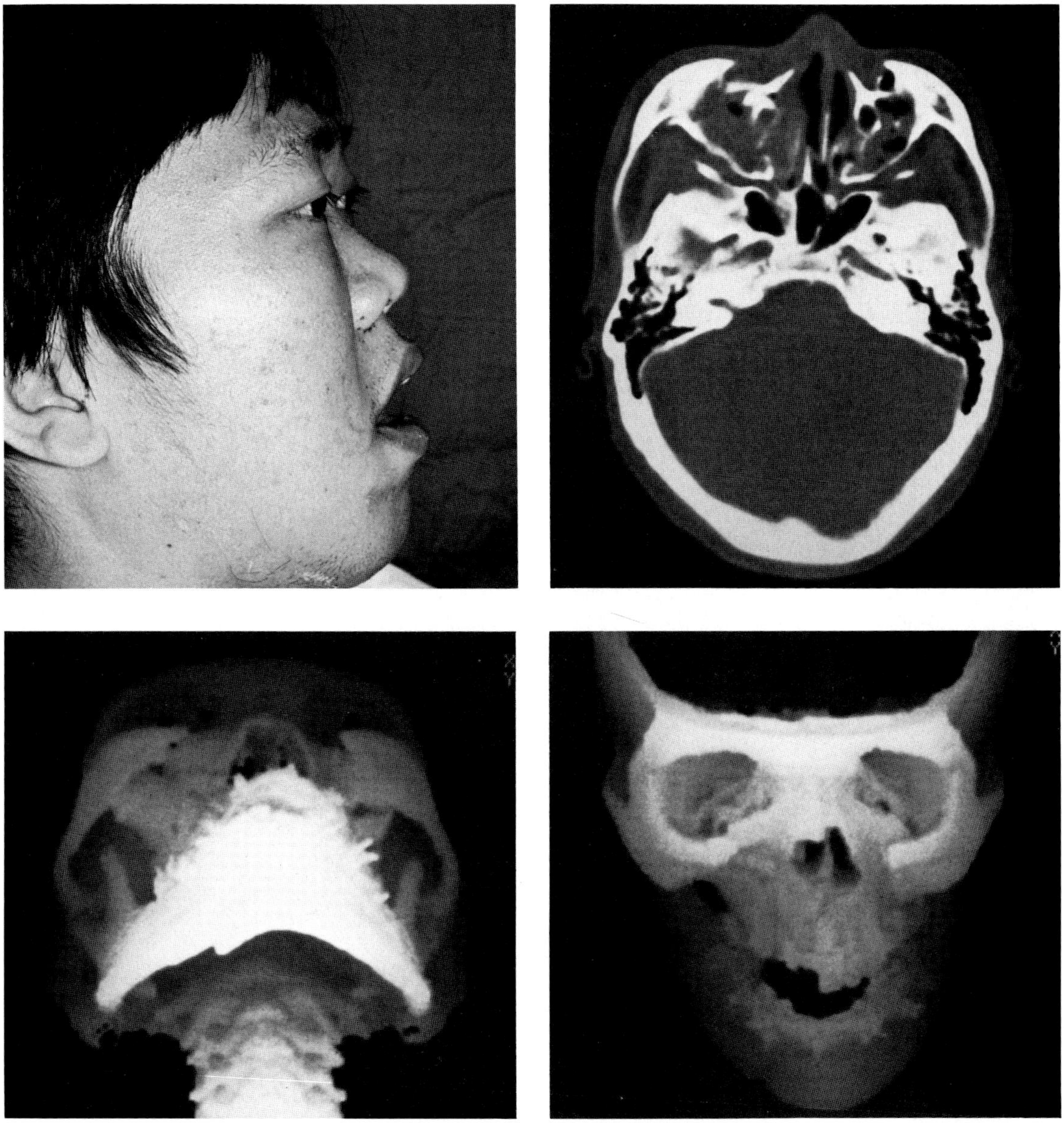

Fig. 9.7. A Severe midfacial flattening is well demonstrated in this Asian patient with a Le Fort II fracture. **B** Zygomatic arches are intact, but the anterior maxillary walls are depressed bilaterally, consistent with a Le Fort II fracture. **C** Parasymphyseal fracture of the mandible and the depressed middle one-third of the face along the Le Fort II fracture line are seen clearly in the chin-up view. **D** When viewed from above, the midfacial disruption with involvement of the medial part of the orbits can be seen, as can the resulting malocclusion.

A B

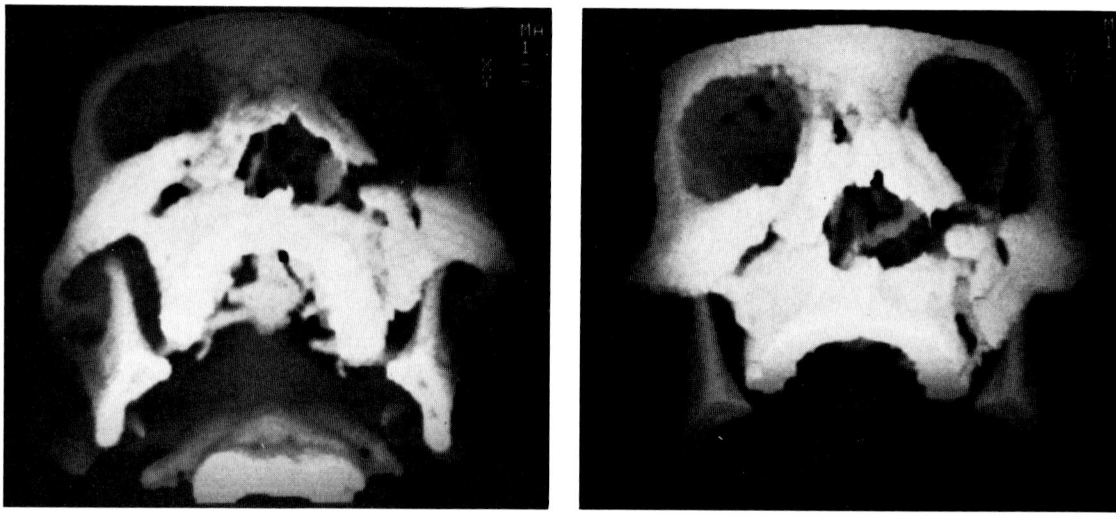

C

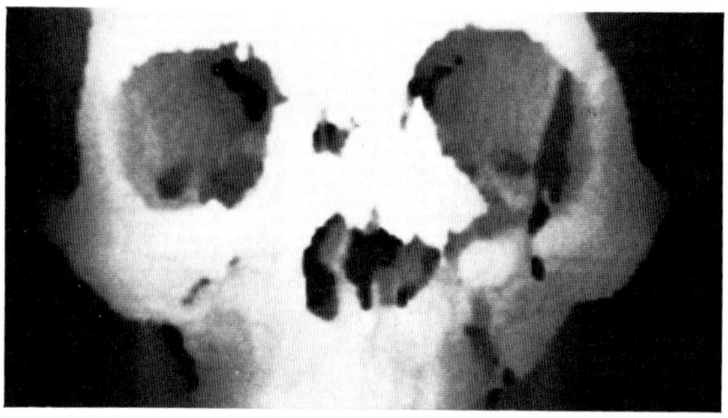

Fig. 9.8. A–C Le Fort II fracture on the right and Le Fort III fracture on the left with disruption of the left lateral orbital wall and buckling of the left medial orbital wall. There is also a Le Fort I fracture. The right zygomaticofrontal complex is the only unfractured area on this face.

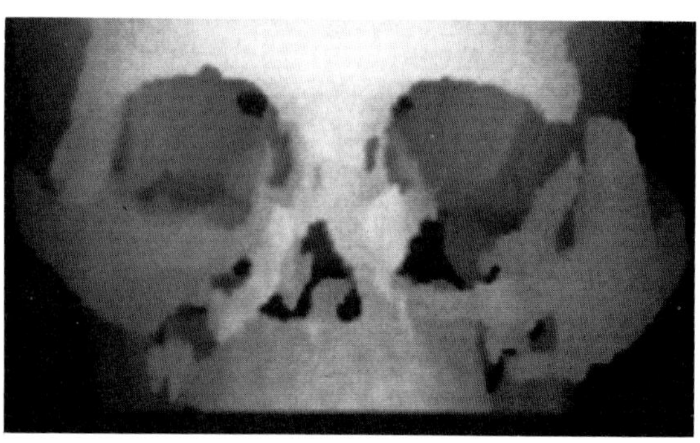

Fig. 9.9. All levels of the midfacial skeleton were involved as a result of an automobile accident. There are bilateral Le Fort I, II, and III fractures.

A B C D

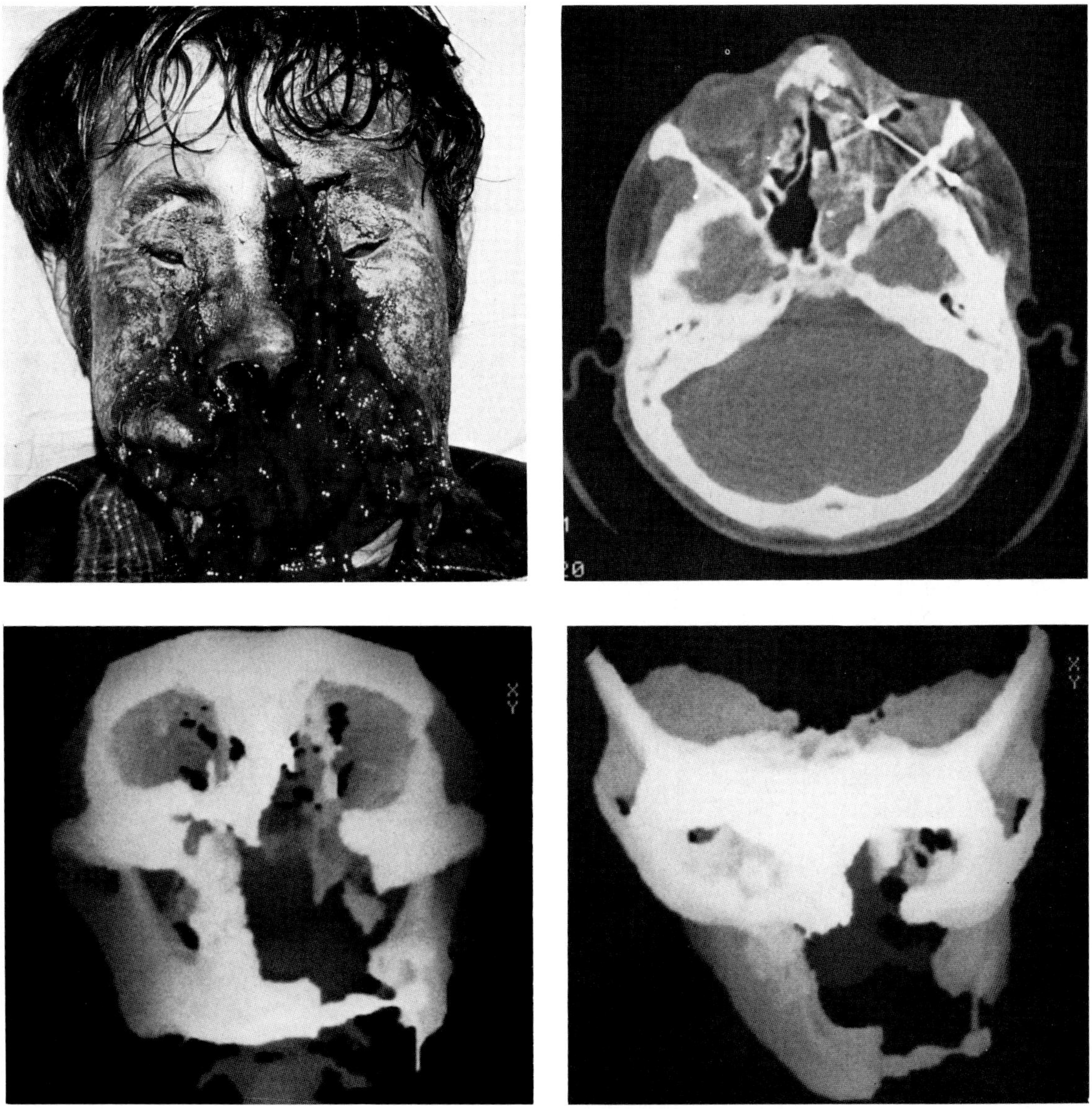

Fig. 9.10. **A** This photograph was taken on admission to hospital of an adult man who sustained a 12-gauge shotgun injury with considerable loss of bone and soft tissue. **B** Radiating artifacts are produced by shotgun pellets. **C** Massive disruption of the left orbit and nasal complex has occurred. There is significant bony loss of the left side of the maxilla, absence of the alveolus, and partial mandibular loss. The connection between the two mandibular fragments is a wire. **D** When viewed from above, the degree of bony deficit of the left orbit, maxilla, and mandible can be clearly seen. The frontal bone has been unaffected.

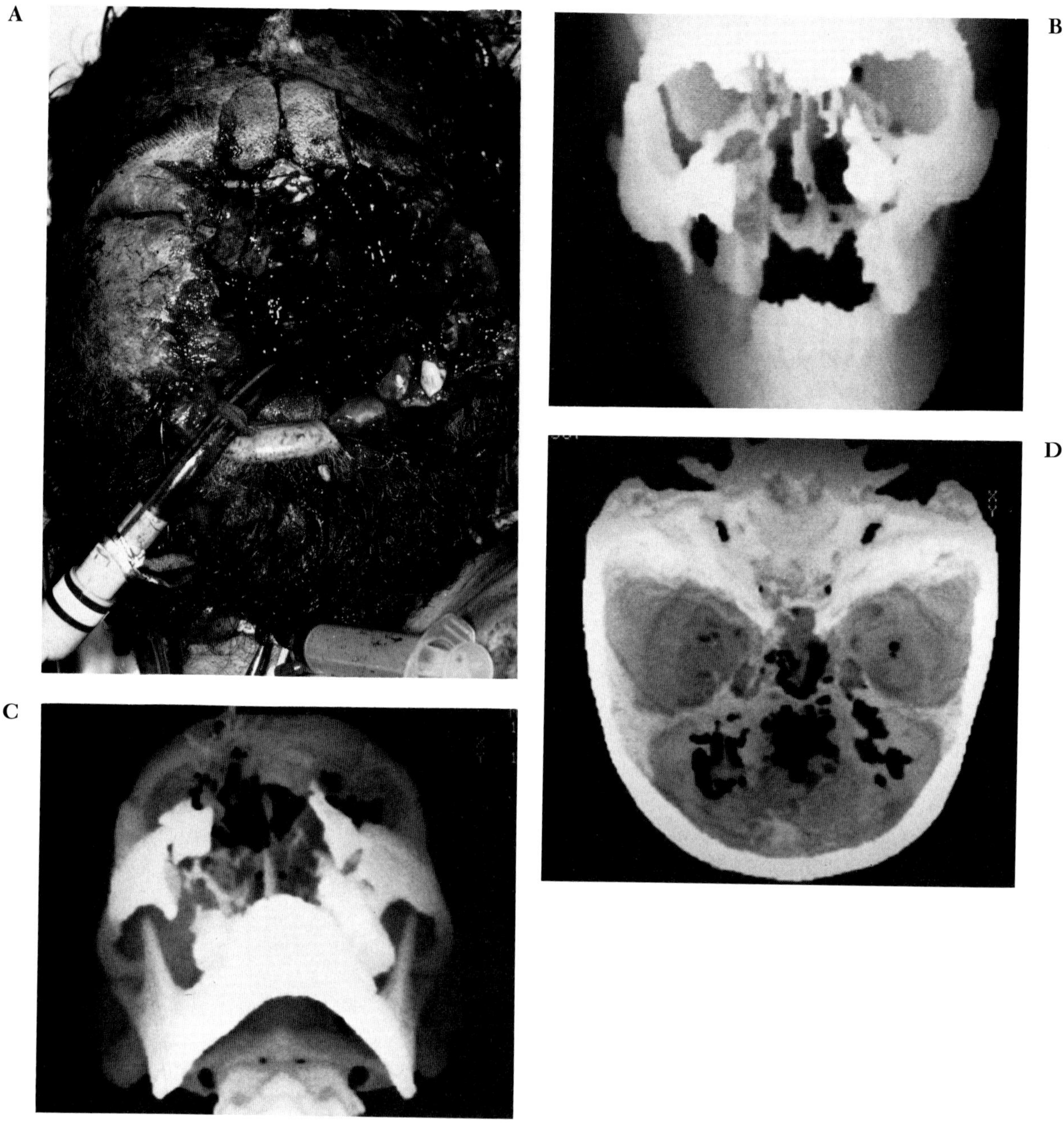

Fig. 9.11. **A** A midline close-range gunshot injury resulted in bilateral blindness and severe frontal lobe trauma. **B** Only remnants of the maxilla remain. They can be seen, through the defect, on the nasal septum and nasal floor. **C** The traumatic defect in the floor of the anterior cranial fossa can be appreciated when viewed from below. **D** Viewed from above, disruption of the anterior skull base is seen to be severe.

A B C

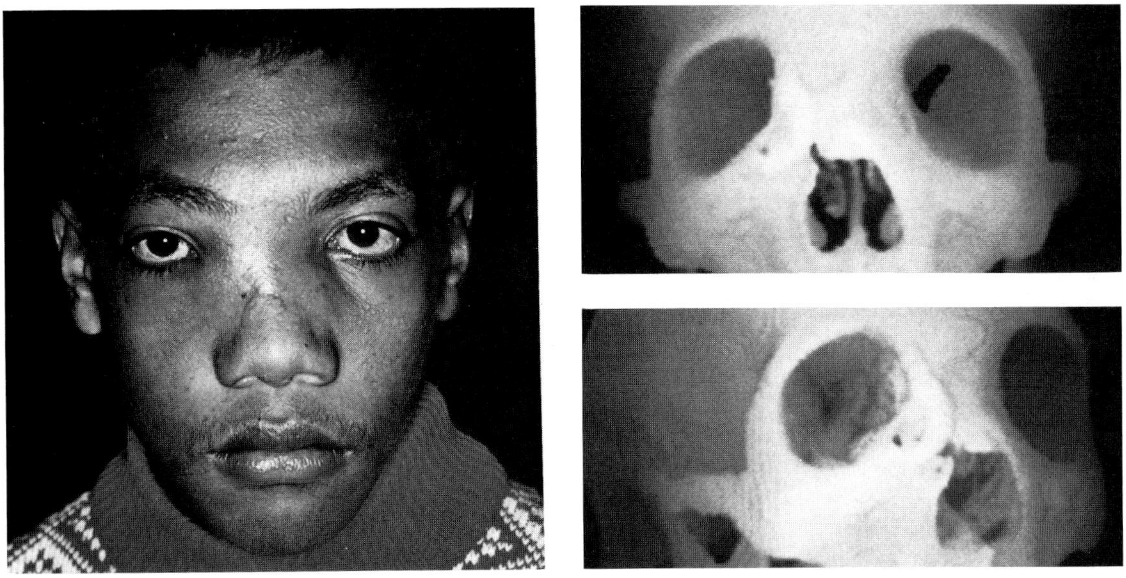

Fig. 9.12. **A** Traumatic telecanthus is present with relatively normal interpupillary distance but widening of the intercanthal region. The defect is due to trauma sustained 7 years prior to the presentation of this 17.5-year-old boy. **B** The disrupted nasoethmoid complex has healed with a widened bony block between the orbits. **C** The healed nasoethmoid fracture has affected the right orbit and the area of the frontal process of the maxilla in the region of the lacrimal bones.

A B C

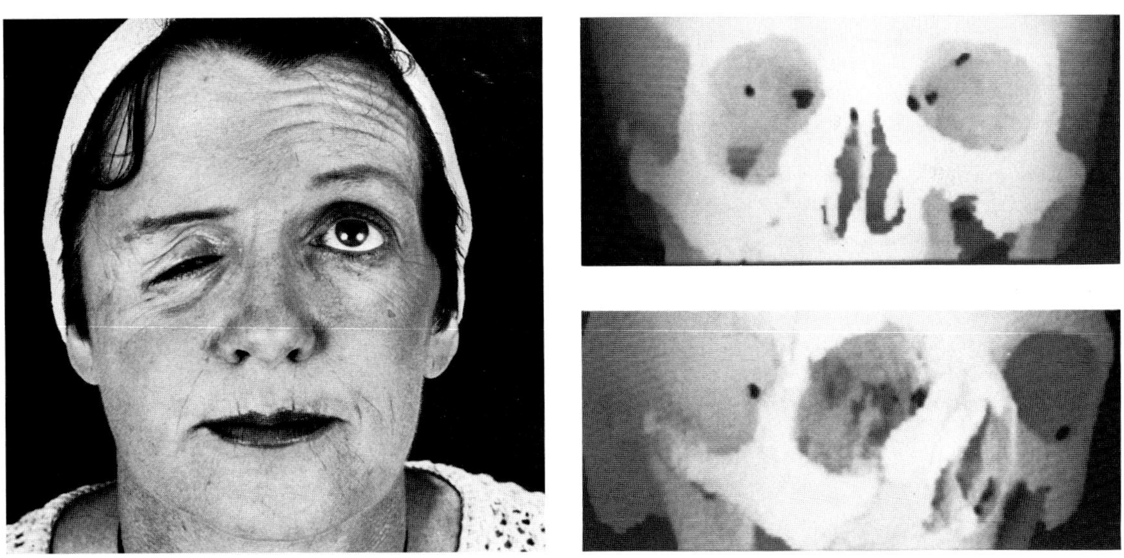

Fig. 9.13. **A** Right orbital disruption resulted from being struck by a brick flying from a truck. **B** The healed zygomatic complex is in a depressed position. The differences in orbital shape and size are obvious, and the zygomatic arch is displaced inferiorly and medially. **C** Healed fractures are demonstrated. Note the difference in right orbital shape from that on the left side.

A B C D

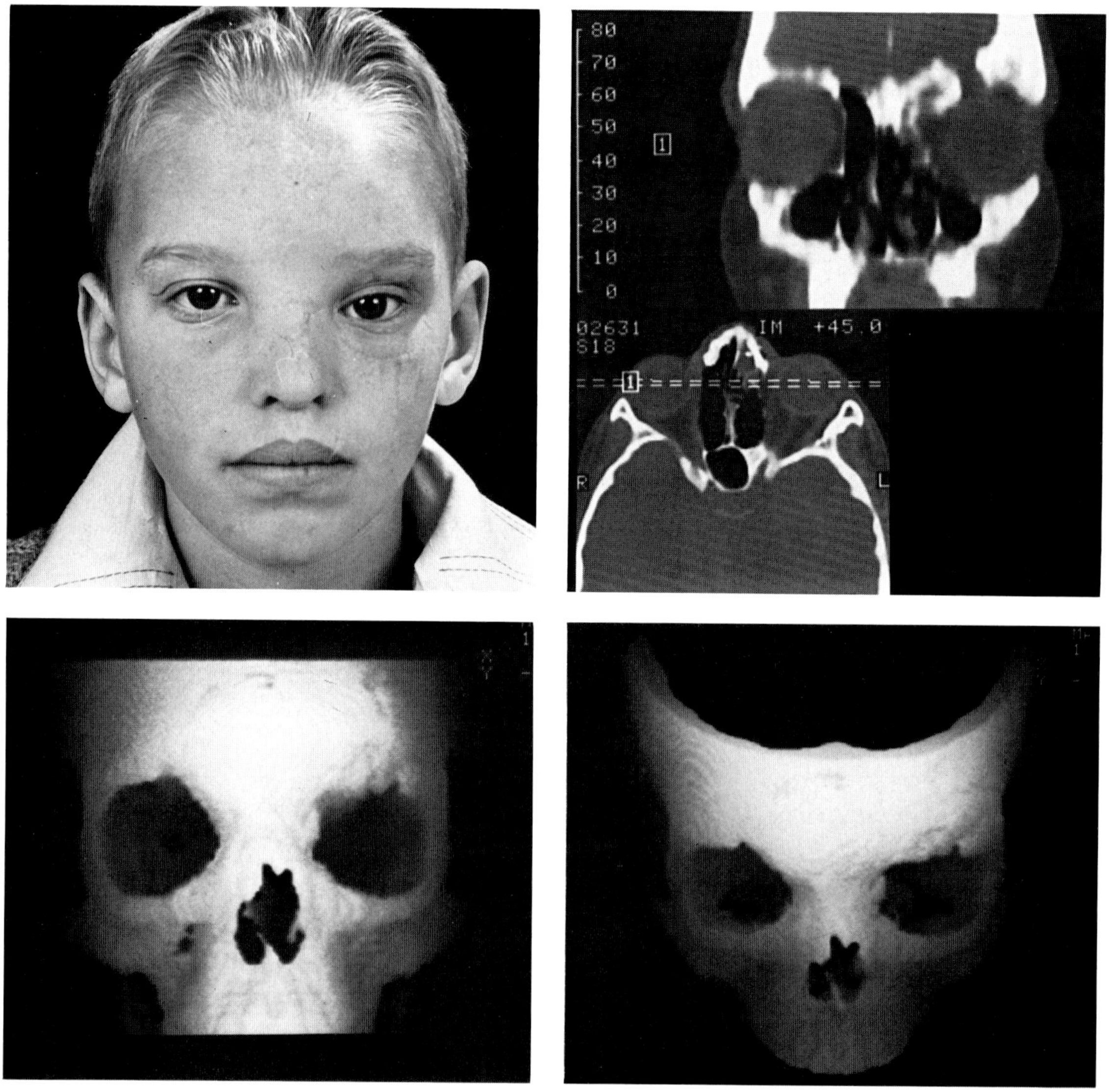

Fig. 9.14. **A** Left orbital dystopia following trauma sustained by being struck by a flying log from a timber truck. The injury resulted in traumatic telecanthus. **B** A defect in the left orbital roof can be seen in the coronal reformatted CT image. **C** Irregularities around the upper left orbital margin are consistent with the previous trauma. **D** There is disruption in the anterior aspect of the medial wall of the left orbit.

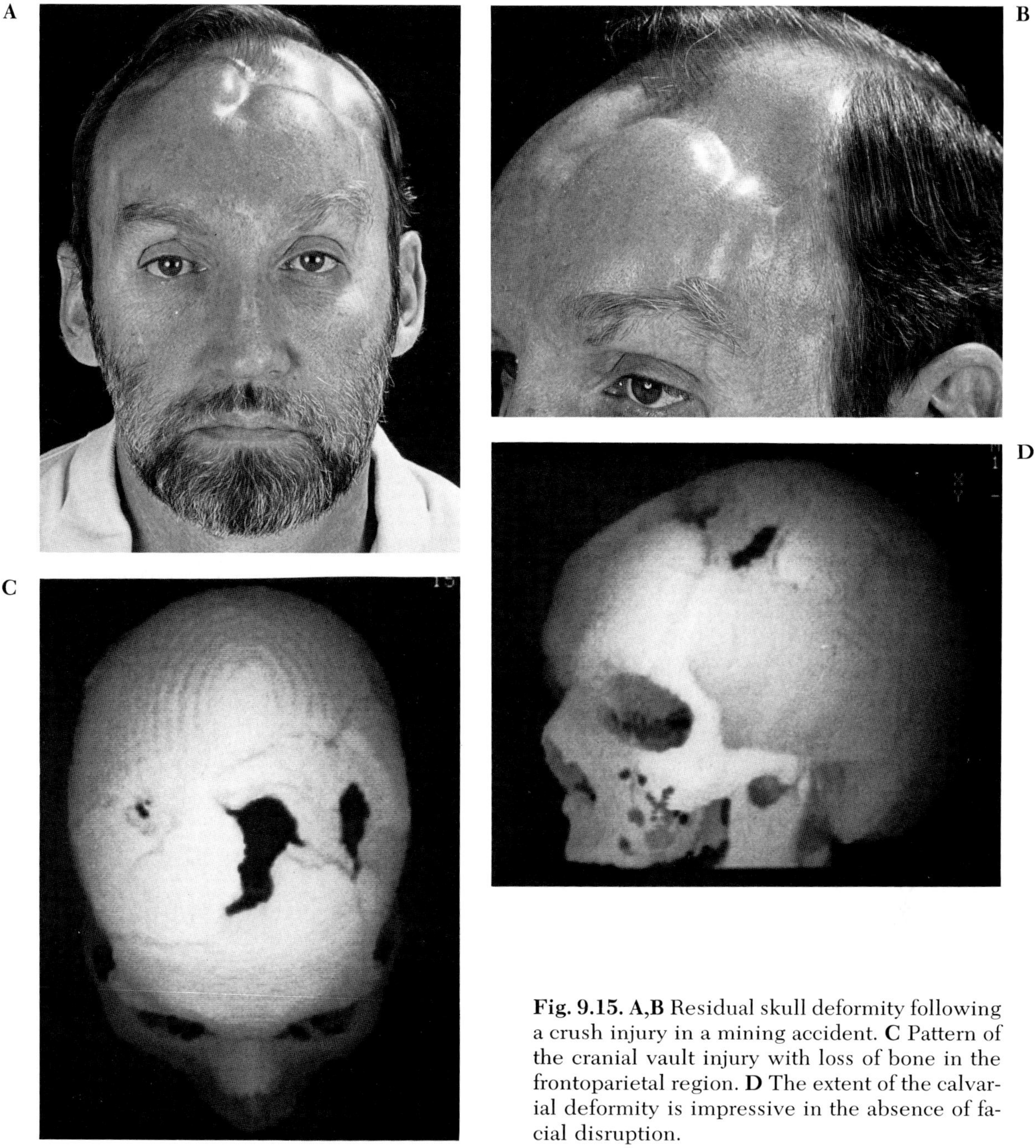

Fig. 9.15. A,B Residual skull deformity following a crush injury in a mining accident. **C** Pattern of the cranial vault injury with loss of bone in the frontoparietal region. **D** The extent of the calvarial deformity is impressive in the absence of facial disruption.

Index